Gender, Power, and Global Social Justice

This book analyses how practitioners can use psychotherapy as a healing mechanism, focusing on the intersection of gender, power, and social justice within the global context.

It begins by interrogating the concept of social justice itself before examining men's and women's issues from biological, sociological, contextual, and ecological perspectives. Each chapter covers individual, couple, and family therapy as well as training and supervising for heterosexual and homosexual individuals from a social justice standpoint.

With a centered and balanced perspective about the impact of gender and power on men's and women's relationships to each other and their ecological contexts, Daneshpour aims to help mental health practitioners privilege client voices, promote justice in gendered relationships, and manage the impact of socio-political issues in therapeutic practice.

Manijeh Daneshpour is distinguished professor of marriage and family therapy and the systemwide couple and family therapy director at Alliant International University in California and a licensed marriage and family therapist with more than two decades of academic, research, and clinical experience.

Gender, Power, and Global Social Justice

The Healing Power of Psychotherapy

Manijeh Daneshpour

Routledge
Taylor & Francis Group

NEW YORK AND LONDON

Cover image: Getty Images

First published 2023
by Routledge
605 Third Avenue, New York, NY 10158

and by Routledge
4 Park Square, Milton Park, Abingdon, Oxon, OX14 4RN

Routledge is an imprint of the Taylor & Francis Group, an informa business

© 2023 Manijeh Daneshpour

ISBN: 9780367542047 (hbk)
ISBN: 9780367542054 (pbk)
ISBN: 9781003088189 (ebk)

DOI: 10.4324/9781003088189

Typeset in Baskerville
by Newgen Publishing UK

To my father for being a philosopher and a critical thinker incredibly ahead of our time and context and to my mother for being a strong role model!

Contents

Acknowledgment

As an academician, researcher, and clinician, I have been supported by many people to strive to work hard, multitask, teach with passion and enthusiasm, become a well-differentiated director and mentor, and an emotionally balanced therapist. Perhaps my secure attachment to my parents is a foundation for my strength and success, or possibly being married to a very kind man for more than three decades and having two strong and sophisticated daughters 14 years apart have contributed to my honest attempt to be a good partner and a loving mother. Perhaps access to financial and emotional resources throughout my childhood and adulthood has helped me to make every effort to develop a solid sense of self.

I would like to thank my father, who was the most significant source of inspiration in my life. When I was new to my feminist thinking and was so proud of my newfound identity, he challenged my thinking, saying that feminist theories are useless in practice unless women become educated and financially independent. He financially and emotionally supported his three daughters to finish their education and start their careers before getting married and told our husbands that our professional identities must be as important as our relational identities. I would like to thank my mother as a very strong role model holding a special place in our journey by keeping all men in her life, including my father, accountable for their deeds toward women while also teaching us how to be supportive partners to our spouses. I am thankful to my older brother, who has always teased me for being short and not as bright as him and also believed in my ability to do well in life. My two sisters, one seven years older and one eight years younger, deserve appreciation because they both taught me how to be the middle child lost in between their strong personalities and also supported and appreciated me in every possible way.

My husband Amir deserves special appreciation since he has been my most stable source of support. We were both undergraduate students in Utah during the Iran-Iraq war with little access to money from our parents from Iran due to the US economic embargo on Iran. He got a physically challenging night shift job at a bakery, not par with his middle-class background. He worked full-time while also going to school to pay our international student tuition to finish our undergraduate degrees. He always says women are as smart as men but need more opportunities to show their skills and talents. I would not have been where I am professionally if not for his unconditional support, love, and sacrifices. Writing this book took all my time and energy for the past two years, primarily because of my demanding and time-consuming administrative and academic responsibilities. Amir took care of all household and family duties with love so I could focus on my writing. I am eternally grateful.

I also owe a lot of gratitude to my daughter, Hoda. She was part of my educational journey and had to sacrifice getting the unconditional attention she deserved while I was busy studying and building a professional career. I owe special thanks to my younger daughter Neda. She had to be super understanding and flexible because I was busy working on papers, traveling to conferences, and seeing clients when I needed to read books to her and play with her. When she was older, I did not go to any extracurricular activities, especially her speech and debates tournaments. She always accepted my apologies and lack of presence with grace and kindness.

This list of acknowledgments can only capture a small fraction of the people who have supported me over the years. I must give special thanks to my professors, supervisors, colleagues, clients, and students who gave me the benefit of doubts and accepted a *Hijabi* Middle Eastern woman to be their student, friend, colleague, therapist, and teacher. They all allowed me to be my authentic self and stay bold, kind, considerate, and not afraid of being wrong, and learn from mistakes made along the way. Thank you all for providing professional learning opportunities and helping me believe in human decency and love. Your contributions to my personal and professional journey were vital. I send my deepest thanks to you all.

At last, the role of gender and power in our everyday interactions are incredibly crucial in how we relate to each other. Thus, advocating for relational and social justice must be central in providing psychotherapy due to our expanding responsibilities. I hope to highlight the critical role of exploring our own positionalities and societal privileges when we engage in relational and social justice advocacy work with men and women and also explore their power and privileges in their relationships. I am profoundly and eternally indebted to everyone who has helped me become a woman with a powerful conviction to social justice, for appreciating men and women and their everyday struggles, and for learning how to do relational and social advocacy work.

A Few Words About Me

I am a cisgender woman from Iran. I grew up in a highly educated middle-class family that perceived gender as a social construct. My parents raised us to believe that women have the capacity and the drive to be as capable as, if not more capable than, men. We were raised in an environment conducive to developing a powerful sense of self, preparing us to see ourselves beyond being women as capable and multidimensional human beings. When I was a child, my father owned a K-12 private school for boys and enrolled me as the only girl in all boys' schools. I finished K-6 with boys, being part of the boys' scout and boys' soccer teams. I often found boys straightforward in their communication but at times insensitive and rude. They showed their frustration loud and clear and without any tact or use of diplomacy. When I switched to an all girls' school for my middle school education, excited to be included among my own kind, I often found girls emotionally available and kind but manipulative and sneaky. It seemed that they needed to be careful and strategize for everything they needed to do or say.

Decades later, my elementary school exposure to boys and middle and high school exposure to girls helped me tremendously as a therapist. I was able to be an emotional container for men's pain and understand their vulnerabilities behind the facade of toughness and being mean and disrespectful to women. I was also able to be the emotional container for women's pain and help them heal the wounds of relational trauma with men. My master's thesis and doctoral dissertation were about the gendered experiences of men and women. Throughout my professional work conducting research, providing couples' therapy, and supervising students, I developed skills in utilizing the axis of gender in addition to generation in working with same-sex and heterosexual couples.

It is worth mentioning that about four decades ago when I immigrated to the US, I was wearing hijab, first based on the simply undeniable destiny that I was born in Iran and my parents were practicing Muslims, and second, I wanted to hold on to my cultural and religious identity. Years later, I realized my developed identity as an educated, capable, confident, liberal, and intellectually bright woman is not as crucial as how others perceived me with my head wrapped in a scarf. I realized that even highly knowledgeable, educated, and liberal people from Eastern and Western cultures could not see me as the whole person beyond the piece of cloth covering my hair. None of these intersectional categories of my identity were intriguing to people, except how perhaps men in my family, especially my Iranian husband, might have somehow oppressed me because I looked like a devout Muslim woman.

Henceforth, when religion was no longer a salient part of my identity, I consciously decided to continue to politically wrap my head with a scarf to stand against the Western hegemony that open-minded and intellectually sophisticated feminists are supposed to look like white women and their hair has to show to be considered a progressive thinker! Thus, when presenting at conferences, teaching classes, attending leadership meetings at the university, or greeting new clients in my office, I routinely explain why I wear hijab and explain my intersectional identities to ease people's level of discomfort about how I look and then work on making a connection.

Over the years, I have noticed that I don't have the luxury of not being attuned to sociocultural contexts because of my physical appearance. I had to become familiar with sociopolitical theories of gender and understand the impact of structural and internalized racism. Through my own, at times harrowing experiences, I have become sensitive and attuned to people's experiences as gendered individuals and understand that our intersectionality and social locations influence our everyday experiences regardless of our level of consciousness.

I have been thinking about writing a book about the sociopolitical aspects of our gendered experiences and how psychotherapy can be a source of healing for our relational wounds for some time. In the classroom, therapy room, and even my own living room, I have seen people's transformation into having a better sense of self and a better sense of agency when they understand their gendered self and advocate for themselves.

As a third-wave feminist, often misunderstood and dismissed simply because of a piece of cloth on my head, I am aware that this book may not get the attention it deserves compared to if it was written by other women who don't share my specific intersectional identities. Nevertheless, my sociopolitical views and clinical and academic backgrounds became deep foundations for the urgency to write this book. I wanted to share sociopolitical and anthropological theories and research about the gendered basis of our interactions and how it has evolved. I also wanted to share my professional knowledge, experience, and expertise, so men and women can learn to understand their gendered selves, honor their relational pain, and be aware of political and cultural issues impacting their everyday experiences. I wanted to challenge psychotherapists to create a safe space for their clients to deal with the agony caused by our genderless, classless, and color-blind approaches to psychotherapy.

Advocating for the most vulnerable is the most ethical part of socially just psychotherapy. In my clinical work, I challenge clients' unfairness and unjust actions and advocate for those with less power, even if they are not part of the therapy process. I interrupt oppressive gendered patterns and challenge the unfair patriarchal hierarchy. I help people with transformative change by providing meaningful and relevant information, tapping into their personal resources, and empowering them to use their sense of agency to challenge themselves and others. I use my knowledge, expertise, and relational skills to help people change their perspectives and become their own agents of change.

Writing this book is a serious attempt to cover gender, power, and global social justice issues, including a balanced perspective about men's and women's relational experiences within the ecological context of different cultures. The current sociopolitical climate in the US and elsewhere and complex issues related to gender, power, and privilege have created a serious void in the psychotherapy field for dealing with men's and women's relational challenges. I firmly believe that we cannot stand by and be neutral in the face of political movements that challenge our progress toward equality and are adversarial to the human vision that underlies psychotherapeutic principles. I believe that therapists are moralists and cannot and should not remain neutral. Thus, we must take the current gender-based challenges seriously and advocate for social justice for heterosexual and homosexual relationships within the therapeutic contexts. We must not accept anything less from ourselves as human beings, relationship experts, and ethical psychotherapists.

Foreword

Academicism, researcher and clinician, Dr. Daneshpour enlightens us about the intersectional challenges of gender, race, religion, class, culture, and nationality – the intersectionality between social inequities, power imbalances, and systemic discrimination. Her goal: relational healing by guiding clinicians to work within the framework of gendered power and relational dynamics.

She encourages mental health practitioners to hear the *client's voice* in their gendered and sociopolitical relationships, and how we can "anti-pathologize their symptoms," the latter a topic I emphasize in my writings.

In her recurring theme of power imbalance, she explains the relationship between patriarchy and violence against women and girls. Internationally, this has led to unequal access to education, health, and security. Worldwide, equality for women and girls has not yet been achieved.

Because women especially are at risk globally due to lower status, few reproductive rights and opportunities for self-sufficiency, the gendered relationships and power dynamics must play a central role between therapist and client, supervisor, and trainee.

The question of whether a therapist can be political is discussed. I found her eighth chapter, about the so-called hard-wired gendering of war and peace especially noteworthy. In the end, Dr. Daneshpour's expansive thesis is about the healing power of psychotherapy.

Pauline Boss, *Professor Emeritus, University of Minnesota.*
Author of The Myth of Closure, *and* Ambiguous Loss,
Harvard University Press, 2000. WW Norton, 2022.
For more, see <www.ambiguousloss.com>

Introduction

Justice refers to the concept of fairness. Social justice manifests fairness in society, including fairness in access to healthcare, employment, housing, quality education, and much more. In the seventeenth century, after the Industrial Revolution, social justice was applied to economics. Now, however, social justice applies to race and gender, issues related to human rights, access to resources, participation of the marginalized in society, and equity for all regardless of their cultural and racial backgrounds. Social justice can't be achieved without equity. Equity is different from equality in that equity considers the impact of discrimination and strives for equal outcomes. Racial, class, gender equality, and LGBTQT rights are now among the most critical issues concerning power dynamics in society.

Further, women, power, and social justice seem to be a provocative amalgamation of words. A woman cannot be too rich, thin, or powerful. She had better know how to conceal herself if she is powerful because otherwise, she will pay the price. Accomplished women have been burned at the stake, forced to run out of town, or got overly sexualized because it has been the simplest way to destroy them. On the other hand, there is no question that women have always influenced men in power behind the scenes.

The current research about men and masculinity explores an overdue recognition and appreciation of men as gendered beings. Thus, starting in the 1990s, a new movement to understand the male side of gender and the concept of masculinity has begun in the UK and US focusing on the concerns about the increase in male unemployment, the decrease in the percentage of men in higher education, and issues related to boys' academic performance in schools. In the Beijing Declaration, adopted by the Fourth World Conference on Women in 1995, many governments expressed a desire to advocate for gender equality, knowing that lack of equality makes men and women suffer.

Even though these developments are important and central in advocating for gender equality, discussions about gender continue to focus more on women. When we talk about gender, we mostly mean women because the disadvantages girls and women face are substantially more than those faced by boys and men. However, the inclusion of men in gender work may make the interventions for women more meaningful because women's well-being

DOI: 10.4324/9781003088189-1

may not be enhanced devoid of involving men. After all, gender is relational and negotiable. Therefore, examining issues related to gender, especially those disadvantaging women, necessitates understanding the experiences and perceptions of both women and men. To understand men, we must appreciate masculinity, examining what it takes to be a man. Thus, social constructs that govern men's and women's attitudes and conduct in gender relations must be understood to take actions aimed to help women effectively.

There are other important considerations for including both genders in advocating for gender equality. Mainly, gender systems have impacted both men and women. Consequently, generalizing about men's and women's experiences ignores gender-specific imbalances and susceptibilities and within-group dominations and discriminations such as the privileged older women's power over younger or poorer women or the influence of more powerful and influential men over younger or poorer men. Further, globalization, economic disparities, ever-growing scarcity of resources, and social changes have weathered men's traditional role as protectors and providers. These changes have confused men about their masculinity, forcing them to seek affirmation by unsafe sexual practices and intimate and social violence, disturbing men, their partners, families, and society.

Objectives and Origin

This book attempts to focus on the intersection of gender, power, social justice within the global context, and the healing power of psychotherapy, aiming to create a balanced perspective about the relational dynamics of men and women in heterosexual and homosexual relationships. It aims to cover gender in the global context examining men's and women's issues from the biological, sociological, contextual, and ecological perspectives. It combines these insights with a clinical approach providing readers with tools and skills necessary to provide psychotherapy utilizing critical thinking skills and, ultimately, investigating gendered power from a global perspective to become better helpers and healers.

Further, social justice and psychotherapy represent the intersection between social inequities, relational power imbalances, and systemic societal discrimination. Thus, the book's central aim is to focus on using psychotherapy as a healing mechanism to help us with our gendered experiences within the global context. The goal is to provide guidance for mental health practitioners to learn how to privilege client voices, promote justice in our gendered relationships, and highlight how we can anti-pathologize symptoms and deal with the impact of sociopolitical issues in our therapeutic practice.

Organization of the Book

The book is organized into 12 chapters examining men's and women's issues from the biological, sociological, contextual, and ecological perspectives. It delves into topics such as nature, nurture, masculinity, women's issues, the impact of Western colonization, politics, religion, war, violence, work, as well as race and class and their impact on our everyday gendered interactions.

Chapter 1," Gender, Nature, Nurture," attempts to define gender, summarize research on gender differences, examine the nature of masculinity and femininity, describe theories of gender, and present a model that argues that nature and nurture are intertwined and complex. The discourses are based on the scientific findings on gender differences, similarities, and variations in sexuality, cognitive abilities, and social behaviors. It also tries to identify, discuss, and clarify some crucial issues for psychotherapists explaining how gender impacts our everyday relationships. The main goal is to provide guidance and insights which can assist clinicians in working within the framework of gendered power and relational dynamics to provide relational healing.

Chapter 2, "Masculinity in Global Contexts," discusses how gender is about relationships of desire and power in a global context and must be examined from both sides. In understanding gender inequalities, it is critical to examine the more privileged group as well as the less privileged. This chapter examines men's gender practices and the ways the gender order defines, positions, empowers, and constrains men cross-culturally. It discusses the gender positions of White men in industrial societies as well as men of color in other cultures. It explores what society constructs for men who may not correspond precisely with what men actually are, or desire to be, or what they actually do. It attempts to identify, discuss, and clarify some important concepts for mental health professionals working with heterosexual and homosexual men within the context of couple and family relationships. It also provides guidance to assist clinicians in working within the framework of gendered power and relational dynamics.

Chapter 3, "Women's Rights in Global Contexts," examines women's issues from an international perspective because the decisions, concepts, and agendas that are being set at the international level shape the conditions of women's lives in societies and families. Those agendas and decisions determine the policies and situations we all live in. There is no longer any part of the world that is unaffected by the global economy, by global culture, and by the kinds of decisions that are being made internationally. Yet, in almost all those arenas, women are underrepresented, if represented at all. Across the globe, women have fewer prospects for economic participation than men. They struggle for equal access to education, must deal with more significant health and security threats, and to a lesser extent, political representation.

On the other hand, empowered women and girls contribute to the health and productivity of their families, communities, and countries, creating a ripple effect that benefits everyone. However, within the Western cultural discourse, women from Eastern cultures are believed to be suffering more and are in need of more support and resources, which masks the fundamental issues related to all women's struggles cross-culturally. This chapter attempts to examine women's relational issues beyond specific borders and cultures and redefine how psychotherapy can have healing power for women in any cultural context. The main goal is to provide guidance and insights which can assist clinicians in working within the framework of gendered power and relational dynamics for women in heterosexual and homosexual relationships.

Chapter 4, "The Impact of Colonization on Global Social Justice," delves into an examination of the nineteenth century as an era of worldwide social change challenging the religious and social basis of all societies. This was when European colonial powers formed the political and economic ideological framework influencing the world and making European men the most direct agents of empires. It discusses how male theorists of imperialism and postcolonialism have seldom felt moved to explore the gendered dynamics of the subject, even though it was White men who operated the merchant ships and wielded the rifles of the colonial armies. It was White men who owned and oversaw the mines and slave plantations, and it was White men who commanded the global flows of capital and rubber-stamped the laws of the imperial bureaucracies. Further, it discusses how even though White, European men, by the close of the nineteenth century, owned and managed 85 percent of the earth's surface, the crucial but concealed relation between gender and imperialism, until very recently, have been unacknowledged or shrugged off as a grim reality of nature. This chapter also discusses how the areas to undergo a radical transformation in the world have been relations between the sexes and family issues and examines all the changes and challenges related to colonial/postcolonial matters to create a context for gendered families' problems. It provides psychotherapeutic guidance and insights to men and women who are impacted by colonial and postcolonial discourses.

Chapter 5, "Gender and Religion," examines gender inequality due to the religious norms which predominate in all societies. It discusses the vital role of religion in the cultural life of all people and how it is deeply rooted in people's everyday experiences and impacts societies' socioeconomic and political direction. In fact, for most social geographic investigations, religion may now be a more critical variable than race or ethnicity. Furthermore, the chapter discusses how the status of women in society is an outcome of the interpretation of religious texts, and the role of religion continues to be complex and varies across time and space. The central premise is that everyone benefits from gender equality, and women's liberation is an essential consideration for the economic, social, and democratic progress of the world's regions and the development of human society. It further evaluates the influences of institutional norms, as well as culture and tradition, which are both largely determined by religion. This chapter also discusses how psychotherapy can have healing power for men and women impacted by the globally religious doctrine of gender relations.

Chapter 6, "Gender and Politics," aims to map out some significant current politics and gender research concepts. The most central ideas in political science and gender and politics research, including democracy, representation, the welfare state, governance, development, gender ideology, intersectionality, and women's movements/feminism, are covered. Further, this chapter covers political science research and the feminist-oriented study of gender to identify the gender-specific patterns of politics and the often inherently gender-biased nature of political science analysis. It also discusses how psychotherapy can have healing power for men and women impacted by local political issues that influence their gendered relationships.

Chapter 7, "Gender, Race, and Class," discusses the complicated interconnection between gender, race, and class, reflecting on the transformations and their profound relationships. These connections reveal the complexity of social relations occurring in contradictory ways to generate a system of race, color, gender, sexual, and class oppression. Within this conceptual frame of multiplicity, the continuation of exclusion, economic exploitation, and state violence must be understood. This chapter further examines the gender dimension as the key. This is because women are at the center of the global economy, whose labor is used to enrich the economy of the elite. The same women also do the socially reproductive work of the world – cleaning, cooking, caring, and unpaid labor. In the meantime, the super-exploitation of men of color goes unnamed and unchecked. Psychotherapy can help people of color articulate anti-sexist, anti-racist, anti-imperialist, anti-capitalist, and anti-homophobic politics. This chapter explains that gender, race, and class do not exist in separate spheres. Instead, they are all interconnected and have a strong and, at times, contradictory relationship to each other. A fundamental assertion of this chapter is that colonialism and the creation of racial categories were essential parts of Western industrial modernity, which became central to the self-definition of the middle class. In addition, racial categories became the source of justification for policing the dangerous classes like the working class, the Irish, Jews, prostitutes, feminists, gays, lesbians, criminals, the rebellious groups, etc. The chapter discusses how psychotherapy can have healing power for men and women of color impacted by the complexity of the interconnection between gender, race, and class influencing their gendered relationships.

Chapter 8, "Gender and War," discusses the consistency of the role of gender in war across all known human societies. It helps readers understand the highly charged debates over the hardwiring of gender traits that associate men with war and women with peace and clear the way for serious consideration of the co-contribution of gender and war. The most significant contribution of this chapter is to show gender to be ontologically enmeshed in combat, which means it is challenging to do war without doing gender and vice versa. This argument is not new. Many feminists have made this point before. However, what is new in this chapter, is evidence from diverse disciplines, to build bridges between feminist, constructivist, and poststructuralist approaches in discussing how gender and war are related. Cultural construction and gendered codes of domination carry the main weight in this argument. The chapter also outlines how psychotherapy can have healing power for men and women impacted by the complexity of war, related to cultural constructions and sexual and economic dominations influencing their gendered relationships.

Chapter 9, "Gender and Violence," examines how gender-based violence arises from the patriarchal system, which has exerted control over women's lives since ancient times. The World Health Organization (WHO) data exposes us to the sad reality that one in every five women has been either physically or sexually abused at some point in their lives. Globally women live in societies mainly characterized by violence against women, affecting their productivity at homes, communities, and places of work. The chapter offers some guidance about how psychotherapy can have healing power for men and women impacted by the power and control dynamics that generate a different source of violence in the relationship.

Chapter 10, "Gender and Work," delves into how work plays a significant role in shaping power and status for both women and men. Work causes gender inequalities in the division of everyday jobs, and women often are not awarded the same prospects as men, regardless of nations' income, developed or developing status. Even though, over the years, some aspects of women's lives and access to opportunities have expanded, their prospects for growth in economics and political areas are still clearly limited. Extensive research about gender roles and stereotyping reveals that all cultures allocate different roles to men and women and have different expectations of both genders. Even though there is not a considerable difference between men's and women's global unemployment rates, the rate for women is consistently somewhat higher than the men. We have witnessed some progress in recent years, but inequality remains across the three main dimensions of work outside the home, the types of work men and women do, and the comparative pay they collect. Labor force participation is often seen as the prime indicator of changes in women's status.

Nevertheless, gender inequality creates an unfair division of power, resources, and privileges for women in the private sphere, family relationships, and public patriarchy. The chapter discusses these work-related discrepancies' impacts on men and women globally. It also outlines how psychotherapy can have healing power for men and women impacted by the unfairness of work and family balance in their relationship.

Chapter 11, "Awareness of Intersectionality and Self of the Therapist in Training and Supervision," examines power dynamics in all gendered relationships, as a culturally defined set of perceptions, impacting females' and males' behavior, that changes across cultures and time and varies based on power dynamics in every relationship. Furthermore, the strong effect of race, racism, and other sociopolitical factors, as well as the person of the therapist throughout the supervision process, are examined.

Chapter 12, "Conclusion," argues that gender appears to play a central role in psychotherapy as in other domains of life. Thus, systematic influences of gendered relationships need to be considered in all aspects of our lives. The modern and postmodern positions on reality and knowledge should create an ecological context for psychotherapists working with men and women in heterosexual and homosexual relationships and from different cultural contexts. This combination makes the potential for drawing widely from the whole field of psychotherapy to heal the wounds of our gendered relationships. This chapter summarizes the book's central thesis. It concludes that the evolving relationship between clients and psychotherapists must be based on more congruent, object-adequate, encompassing, holding, shared, emotionally safe, conscious, just, provisional, and hopeful dynamics.

1   Gender, Nature, Nurture

Introduction

Gender is deemed as a range of characteristics distinguishing between masculinity and femininity. These characteristics may include biological sex such as the state of being male, female, or an intersex variation, sex-based social structures such as gender roles, or gender identity. Most cultures use a gender binary with only two genders (boys/men and girls/women). All others fall under the umbrella term non-binary or genderqueer. Various cultures have long recognized members outside of the rigid boundaries of the biological binary. Historians have written about people who were neither men nor women for centuries. Many of these individuals have alternative identities, such as *hijras* in South Asia, *kathoeys* in Thailand, and *muxes* in Mexico, who identify as non-gendered people (Scobey-Thal, 2014).

The concept of gender is recent in human history. It has only been utilized in the studies of human relationships in humanities and social sciences for the past few decades (Coltrane & Adams, 2008; Meyerowitz, 2008). The term gender started to move toward it being a malleable cultural construct in the 1950s and 1960s. John Money, a sexologist, introduced the terminological distinction between biological sex and gender as a role in 1955 (Haig, 2004). Analysis of more than 30 million academic article titles from 1945–2001 showed that the uses of the term "gender" were much rarer than uses of the term "sex," which was often used as a grammatical category early in this period (Haig, 2004). Starting in the 1970s, feminist scholars adopted the term *gender* to make a distinction between "socially constructed" aspects of male-female differences (gender) from "biologically determined" aspects (sex). In this way, gender refers to men's and women's and nonbinary roles and responsibilities created in our families, societies, and cultures in heterosexual and same-gender relationships.

Further, the concept of gender also includes the cultural expectations concerning the characteristics, capacities, and expected behaviors of what is considered feminine and masculine. Social differentiation systems such as political status, class, ethnicity, physical and mental disability, and age modify gender roles. Analyzing and challenging the static use of the concept of gender

DOI: 10.4324/9781003088189-2

is extremely important because when applied to social analysis, it reveals how women's subordination and men's domination are socially constructed. As such, the subordination can be changed or ended since it is not biologically predetermined or fixed forever (UNESCO's Gender Mainstreaming Implementation Framework, 2003).

The following assumptions are the core of my understanding and the basis for all my discussions of the construct of gender in this book:

- Gender roles define the relationship between men, women, and nonbinary individuals. It is also about people's interests, roles, and positions in families and societies.
- Gender roles should focus on people's welfare related to discrimination, needs, equity and equality, empowerment, and gender-based policies.
- Gender defines the varied and complex arrangements between men, women, and nonbinary individuals, encompassing the organization and reproduction of the sexual division of labor and cultural definitions of femininity and masculinity.
- Gender roles are determined by the conception of tasks, functions, and roles attributed to women, men, and nonbinary individuals in society in public and private lives.
- Gender identity is not determined at birth. As the child matures, physiological and social factors contribute to the early establishment of a core identity modified and expanded by social factors. Thus, gender identity develops through social reinforcement and language.
- Gender is always part of the larger sociocultural context. Gender indicates what social attributes and opportunities are associated with being male and female and what society expects, allows, and values in a woman, man, or nonbinary person in a given context. There are disparities and inequalities between women and men in decision-making opportunities, responsibilities assigned, activities undertaken, and gaining access and controlling resources in most societies. Other essential criteria for socio-cultural analysis include class, race, poverty level, ethnic group, and age.

The Nature of Masculinity and Femininity

Humans have organized social life around gender in fundamental ways. Even before a child is born and onward, parents and society assume that boys and girls are very different and treat them accordingly. The first wave of feminists in the 1970s seemed to embrace the notion of gender as a social construct, which creates differentiation between men and women in areas such as work, family life, roles, and responsibilities. Ann Oakley's text, *Sex, Gender and Society* (1974), created an essential foundation for further exploration of the construction of gender. She examines how Western cultures seem to exaggerate gender differences and create a culture around the notion of gender differences. It appears that few factors influence people's lives from birth to death as much as sex or gender. Gender is central from the insignificant to the most profound aspects of our lives. Often, things are defined based on gender when they can be characterized as either masculine or feminine and reveal patterns of differences by gender. In fact, "masculinity" and "femininity" describe gender identities and what it means to be a man, woman, or nonbinary person in a given society.

Our social relationships are culturally constructed and ultimately impacted by our perception of masculine and feminine. That is how a particular culture uses explicit notions of defining masculine and feminine (Ashraf, 2018). We turn to nature by using biology, differences in the body's structure, hormones, muscles, and genes to show how they impact our differences. We turn to different aspects of our relationship with others and societal expectations to show how nurture influences our differences. Sylvia Walby (1990) identified two main and broad approaches to the subjective understanding of gender socialization theory and discourse analysis.

Socialization theory explains masculine and feminine identities as part of a socialization process beginning in childhood with masculine behavior being illustrated by assertiveness, action-orientedness, and forcefulness, whereas feminine is the set of behaviors shown by passivity, being cooperative, and gentleness. Based on this approach, preparation and socialization for one or the other gender attributes start right at birth. Toys, parental interactions, activities, language, television programming, and reading material are geared to suit the specific gender. These patterns continue throughout our adult lives through images of women as sexually attractive and glamorous and men as successful and influential. The socialization theory stresses reinforcing the sexual division of labor by the family, media, and the entire education system to create and perpetuate masculine and feminine subjects. Walby (1990) discusses the limitation of this approach because of its inability to realize that gendered culture is constructed in all areas of social life and not just media, family, and education.

Walby (1990) prefers a discourse analysis approach stating that gendered subjectivity is created continuously and in all of our interactions. They do not happen in specific sites or places, and they are not just about our early childhood experiences or sexuality. Therefore, Walby claims that changing gendered relations in all areas is the basis for generating new norms of femininities and masculinities. The struggles over these norms contribute to our understanding of what needs to change. While there have been significant changes in what is considered masculine or feminine, the fact is that the dichotomy still persists (Ashraf, 2018; Lindqvist *et al.*, 2021). It seems like the notion of femininity is no longer limited to the domestic sphere but located in a far wider arena. However, most societies have moved away from the contextual justification of differences in masculinity and femininity to a more dangerous approach denying the extent of gender inequality because women are no longer explicitly kept out of certain spheres of life. Supposedly there are no barriers preventing women from fully engaging in society, but the facts prove that this is far from the truth.

Theories of Gender Development

Four theories of gender development are the biological, the behavioral, the cognitive, and the psychoanalytic feminism approaches.

Biological – this approach characterizes the gender differences to biological differences embedded in the chromosomes. Human beings have 23 chromosomes, referred to as sex chromosomes, with the female chromosome being XX and the male chromosome being XY. According to biological theory, the behavioral differences between boys and girls are determined by the differences in chromosomes (X/Y) and hormones (testosterone). For instance, the mortality rate for men is higher than women since the XY chromosomal makeup is less stable than XX, and men are more aggressive in almost all cultures, which links the androgen hormones to disruptive and aggressive behaviors. Androgen hormones are also related to male characteristics, with testosterone being the most important androgen.

On the other hand, the XX chromosomal makeup and estrogen seem to make women less vulnerable to physical problems, so women live longer (Mahtab, 2015). Thus, the biological approach suggests that there should not be a distinction between sex and gender since the biological factors – hormones and chromosomes – create gendered behavior. According to Obi (2018), females exposed to high androgens prenatally tend to be more physically active, while the absence or low levels of androgens lead to a less active lifestyle. The study states that the biological process highly contributes to the development of gender roles. However, the cultural differences, cognitive processes, and sex stereotypes that will impact all biological factors cannot be ignored.

Behavioral – while the biological approach claims that nature is the most impactful factor for the development of gender roles, the behavioral approach claims that nurture highly impacts the development of gender and that our behavior and personality are products of our learning environment. Behaviorists highlight the importance of reinforcement and the significance of other variables like social context, observation, and modeling. Thus, the process of learning begins with individuals learning through observation, with the mental states being a central part of this process. However, the behavioral theory asserts that a change in behavior does not always happen when something is learned. The external, mainly environmental reinforcement, influences learning and behavior as it is perceived as a form of internal rewards like pride, satisfaction, and a sense of accomplishment (Obi, 2018).

Cognitive – this approach focuses on thinking and perception as the most critical factors in learning. It states that the way we think determines how we perceive the world, and this perception would affect the way we behave or act. Our mental schema, social experience, and environment shape our gender role behaviors. The cognitive theory states that as children grow up, they gradually develop an organized set of beliefs about the sexes and a strong sense of consciousness about the sex role expectations. Thus, girls and boys learn that they are different and expected to behave like others from their sex group. The most central theme we extract from research on gender socialization is that because boys and girls are treated differently, and their learning environments are different, they develop different needs, wants, desires, skills, and temperaments. Thus, they become vastly different from each other and, interestingly enough, rarely question why they are different or how they ended up being so different. This is explained by the concept of self-fulfilling prophecy, with boys and girls thinking they are supposed to be different. Then, society treats them differently and gives them different developmental opportunities. This continuous and consistent differential treatment stimulates certain behaviors and self-images and reconstructs the predetermined cultural stereotypes about gender. This unending process repeats itself over and over across the generations, so even though they are re-created and modified, they seem natural and impermeable to changes (Haralambos & Holborn, 2014).

Psychoanalytic/Psychodynamic – Freud believed that gender identity in children develops from early, strong but unconscious sexual urges. Between the ages of three and five years, children go through "the phallic stage" and develop strong sexual desires toward the parent of the opposite sex. Therefore, the child becomes jealous of the same-sex parent. Still, it gets resolved by the child becoming fearful of the desires and completely identifying with the same-sex parent, and imitating the same behavior. In this process, according to Freud, the role of both parents in a child's gender development is highly critical, and children raised by one parent would have a much weaker sense of gender identity. He further argues that a boy brought up by a mother without a father would most likely be a homosexual.

Deleuze and Guattari (1983, 1987) and Irigaray (1984, 1985a, 1985b, 2008) criticize Freud and psychoanalysis, offering groundbreaking perspectives. Their ideas help challenge psychoanalysis's way of complicating the man/woman binary production discussing the body, desire, differences, politics, and a sense of becoming. Although Freud's view is problematic for feminism in its resolution, it provides an excellent description of the "othering" of women and their "subordinate and suppressed" role in society. Deleuze and Guattari specifically focus on integrating sexual differences that have been viewed as oppositional, invisible, or the same in phallocentrism. Thus, in discussing the topic of sexual difference, we need to continuously pay attention to the fact that at least two sexes exist, and their feelings, interests, desires, and thoughts should be fully expressed and not repressed. In this sense, Deleuze and Guattari see an abundance of sexes. They suggest that it is impossible to reduce these differences and challenge the psychoanalysis perspective on the binary notion of men and women.

Furthermore, Horney stated that females' envy for males is symbolic and arises from their desire to attain men's higher position in society (Obi, 2018). Men also envy women's ability to reproduce and fight to have more achievements to compensate for this deficiency. Horney also argued that women's sense of inferiority does not arise because of their apparent physical inferiority. The way men behave combined with masculine societal bias infuriates women (Obi, 2018).

Theories of Gender Stratification

Gender stratification examines the significant impact of gender on the power dynamics in societies. Three approaches attempt to explain these different perspectives: the functionalist, conflict, and feminist perspectives.

The functionalist perspective: this approach is based on the structural-functionalist theory, assuming that the society has a stable, organized system in which people's values, beliefs, and behavioral expectations are the same. According to this approach, societies are comprised of interrelated parts, with each part preferably serving a function by contributing to society's general stability. The specific social structures in societies are needed because they are fundamental to societal survival. These institutions consist of the family, educational systems, government, religion, and the financial system. If any of these institutions are negatively altered, other parts are impacted, and the whole system cannot perform appropriately (Kendall, 2003).

The main interest for functionalists, then, is social stability, and the family is a fundamental institution to maintain this stability. Thus, the functionalists insist that gender stratifications are essential for preserving stable families, which in turn protect stable societies. Talcott Parsons, the leading theorist for this approach, states that women instinctively adopt the expressive and emotionally empathetic role. Men naturally take the active and practical role, perfectly and harmoniously complementing each other. Parsons believed that the reason it is so vital for women to continue to have the expressive role is to allow men to have the freedom to perform instrumental tasks. The same is true for women. Thus, women need to attach themselves to the family as wives, mothers, and domestic leaders, while men should perform all the occupational duties in society (Schaefer, 2005).

According to this approach, traditional gender-specific roles are central for individuals and the social order because family life is impacted when the gender role hierarchy changes. This is important because women carry the expressive role of socializing children. When they don't play this role well, society's moral foundation deteriorates, contributing to higher crime rates, violence, and drug abuse. This perspective attempts to prove the centrality of the traditional division of labor between men and women as the natural order for the universe.

The functionalist perspective has been criticized for insisting that gendered division of labor is natural and must be accepted regardless of men's and women's personal preferences. We now know that this claim does not have a fundamental scientific basis, as we see more women being successful in taking up instrumental roles and more men taking on the expressive roles. Further, this perspective does not consider that societies are structured to give more educational and occupational opportunities to men and not take the underlying power relations between men and women seriously or equally value men and women's contributions into consideration (Kendall, 2003).

The conflict perspective – this perspective puts the basis of gender stratification on power, viewing the gendered division of labor as the result of dominance and power over women and societal resources. This approach stresses that men's instrumental abilities are greatly respected and appreciated while women's expressive abilities are completely devalued and unappreciated. Men are basically influential decision-makers and in power both at home and work, disadvantaging women's positions at home and work. More importantly, marriage as an institution is a reflection of male dominance since men of the industrial and capitalist classes established and promoted monogamous marriage. The monogamous marriage is the hallmark of a gendered institution and ensures the paternal lineage of men's descendants, especially their sons, to make sure the right person inherits their wealth (Kendall, 2003). This approach also claims that gender stratification is the natural consequence of private ownership of production and exchange of goods, enabling some men to have ownership and control of property and control and dominate over women. Thus, promoting gender differences reflects the conquest of men over conquered women.

Feminist perspective – this approach uses the conflict theory to further scrutinize the strong reinforcement of gender roles dominating and oppressing women. The feminist perspective seeks to highlight ways cultural norms, societal values, and internalized expectations constrain and control women's behaviors and their relative lack of power (Kendall, 2003). Within the feminist perspectives, there are different perspectives called liberal, radical, and socialist feminism.

Liberal feminists associate gender equality with offering women equal opportunities for growth and development. They also attack male power in oppressing women's lack of equal rights and educational prospects. They believe that gender-role socialization and gender stratification are directly linked. Thus, any effort to solve this problem must begin with focusing on human rights issues and educational attainments. Major efforts must be made in children's homes since it is the first place for their socialization. The schools and the mass media are also essential to correct the distorted and biased gender role biases.

Radical feminism blames male domination as the reason for human oppression, claiming that women's childbearing and child-rearing obligations force them to be dependent on men (Kendall, 2003). More importantly, they believe that society utilizes the media and religion to rationalize and explain the need for male domination and female oppression. Consequently, they promote the idea of eradicating patriarchy and creating complementary institutions that are not gendered and can meet women's needs.

Socialist feminism blames the oppression of women on their two-fold positions as both paid and unpaid laborers in the consumerist and capitalist systems maintaining the dominance of men over women. Socialist feminists advocate for the eradication of capitalism and replacing it with a socialist order to create a context for equal pay for both men and women. Overall, all these perspectives advocate for the importance of considering nurture and our socialization patterns instead of nature and biological bases of behaviors when it comes to gender differences in all societies.

The Complexity of Nature and Nurture

The central realms of human behavior from gender roles, aggression, compassion, love, altruism, egoism, impressionability of our characters, freedom to choose, responsibility, and individuality are all impacted by the nature-nurture debate and continue to be controversial in biology, social sciences, and even in everyday life and politics.

There is still no straightforward method to give a precise and general account of what in humans is 'sheer nature' and what can be attributed to 'sheer nurture.' Furthermore, the central discussion within the context of Darwinism affects the relevance of sociobiological insights into human nature. The 'biological' or 'genetic' determination has come under attack from social sciences and biology. Alternative theories to explain eusociality are being proposed to help us rethink the theoretical foundation of sociobiology (Wilson & Wilson, 2007). Newer theories suggest that the complex interplay between environment, development, the selection at the gene level, the individual level, and even on the group or cultural level shape evolution (Jablonka & Lamb, 2005; Kerr & Godfrey-Smith, 2002; Okasha, 2006; Wilson & Wilson, 2007). This multilevel perspective makes a mono-causal view impossible, leaving the dualistic nature-nurture divide and 'gender determinism' behind.

Given that the first cultural exchanges in human history were many years ago, human 'nature' has in part always been shaped by human 'culture.' Thus, it seems like this contributing and instrumental interconnection or co-evolution was, in fact, crucial in the evolution of mankind. The comparative studies of human and primate cognition (Tomasello, 1999; Tomasello *et al.*, 2005) suggest that humans' ability to develop a complex theory of mind and do things intentionally and jointly with other humans is a unique ability that enables cultural evolution. It is reasonable to assume that 'social cognition' and the challenges of group life, along with the extension of the human brain, increased human dependence on culture. These theories accentuate humans' social or charitable nature and distance humans from the rigid, inflexible, and 'selfish gene' view.

Cultural evolution might then be based on the acquired knowledge of individuals that can be faithfully transmitted and become perfected over generations in an accumulative process. In this view, different traditions can be combined. New ideas can be created not by accidental or random mutations but through thoughtful ideas and intentional advancement, allowing a much 'faster' evolution than biological evolution (Tomasello, 1999).

It remains true that human behavior is not autonomous just because we are shifting the power away from genes to a somewhat more independent understanding of cultural evolution. Cultural determinism can also be a debatable view, just as biological determinism. What is highly appealing is that when we integrate the eccentric capability of people to challenge the status quo, to live out, and to distance himself from his drives, preferences, prejudices, influences, and pre-determinations, we see that nurture and nature are intertwined and continue to be complex and intriguing.

Summary of Gender Research

Gender refers to the "culturally and socially constructed differences between females and males found in the meanings, beliefs, and practices associated with 'femininity and masculinity'" (Kendall, 2003: 339–340). The *Encyclopaedia of Sex and Gender: Culture Society History* (2007) refers to Gender as the condition of being female or male (biological aspect) but also includes the behavioral, cultural, or psychological traits typically associated with one sex into its meanings. McLeod (2004) states that gender refers to the cultural differences expected by society and the culture of men and women according to their sexes.

To summarize these three definitions, gender has a well-defined and robust social inclination, and even though there are physiological differences between men and women, gender is clearly socially determined. Therefore, since gender is directly related to societal perception and expectations, sex does not naturally change from birth, but gender can. McLeod (2004) asserts that "in the past, people tend to have very clear ideas about what was appropriate to each sex and anyone behaving differently was regarded as deviant. Today we accept a lot more diversity and see gender as a continuum" (p. 1).

The central idea in fundamentally all gender studies is that gender is socially constructed in all societies with a clear distinction that there are biological differences between the sexes (such as women's reproductive capabilities). Most societies create norms and values that assign different roles for men and women and then socialize children into these roles. Children observe parents at home from infancy, seeing mothers generally engaging in household chores like cooking, dishwashing, and sweeping, while fathers are typically engaging in more difficult tasks like fixing the car, garage door, and electric appliances. Then the media, school activities, and societal expectations reinforce these early experiences. As the child grows up, they gradually come to realize that women execute less valued and challenging tasks, while men who have more physical strength execute the more difficult and valued tasks. From this process, boys are expected to learn how to be a man, and girls learn how to be a woman; they develop their gender identity perceiving themselves as being either female or male. These stereotypes remain with them, mostly all through their lives, and play a critical role in guiding children through gender roles deemed appropriate in society. Lorber (1994) emphasizes the centrality of the social construction of gender by stating:

> Gender is a human invention, like language, kinship, religion, and technology, like them, gender organizes human social lives in culturally patterned ways. Gender organizes social relations in everyday life as well as in the major social structure, such as social class and the hierarchies of bureaucratic organizations. (p. 6).

Gender Differences in Mental Health Disorders

The gender differences in the manifestation and diagnosis of mental health disorders expand beyond differences in the prevalence of various disorders or their differential time of onset or course. These include several factors that impact the risk level, predispositions, diagnosis, treatment, and adjustment to mental disorder (Afifi, 2007). There are clear gender differences in the prevalence of mental disorders among different age groups. For example, conduct disorder is the most common psychiatric disorder diagnosed during childhood, with the three-time higher prevalence for boys than girls (Afifi, 2007). On the other hand, the prevalence of depression, eating disorders, suicidal ideations, and suicide attempts are higher for girls during the adolescent years. Adolescent boys are more prone to engage in high-risk behaviors and commit suicide more frequently. Women are more prone to developing affective disorders and non-affective psychosis during adulthood, and men are more susceptible to developing substance use disorders and antisocial personality disorders (Afifi, 2007).

Furthermore, men are more likely to develop mental health disorders due to stress, like antisocial disorders and substance abuse. They are socialized to express anger and act out when they feel pressured. On the other hand, women are socialized to express dissatisfaction, anxiety, and restlessness in response to stress. Thus, the higher prevalence of depressive disorders in women is balanced out by higher male alcohol abuse and drug dependency rates. Since mental health professionals do not recognize these gendered base differences at the level that can impact our interventions, men, women, and nonbinary individuals continue to suffer the consequences of this lack of knowledge.

The Healing Power of Psychotherapy

Gender-neutral mental health services will not be effective if societies are interested in reducing risk factors for men, women, and nonbinary individuals. Since the risk factors are gender-specific, and women have lower status and fewer life opportunities in all societies, their lower status can potentially be a dangerous risk for serious mental health problems. An adequate sense of balanced mind and body health requires experiencing self-worth, competence, autonomy, adequate income, and a sense of physical, sexual, and psychological safety and security. The majority of women worldwide are systematically denied many of these resources, impacting their mental health. Thus, it is critical to consider how men and women have different roles and responsibilities, knowledge base, position in society, and different levels of access to health care resources making them more or less vulnerable to developing mental disorders. We also have to improve women's access to resources and teach them how to utilize services. We need to identify factors that can facilitate coping with stress, design public intervention programs, evaluate and strengthen community services to protect and promote women's autonomy and mental health. Health care providers need to be trained to integrate more gender-sensitive services and learn to identify and treat mental illness.

Psychotherapists interested in implementing gender-sensitive philosophy and techniques in their practice have to focus on men and women and nonbinary awareness, empowerment, and identity exploration. They need to examine how both men, women, and nonbinary individuals have internalized social and cultural messages that contribute to the difficulties or pain they are experiencing. Gender-sensitive psychotherapy should first help men and women become aware of how they have been socialized and use coping strategies, avoid diagnosing (unless it is utterly essential) and discuss the impact of social factors on behaviors. If a diagnosis is inevitable, they should involve clients in the process and be conscious and mindful to avoid reinforcing stereotypes (Herlihy & Corey, 2013). It is also critical to look beyond the client's symptoms to understand the impact of environmental and contextual factors and how men and women and nonbinary individuals operate within their environment. For instance, women, men, and nonbinaries who have experienced trauma and abuse have often been labeled with personality disorders even though PTSD is the most appropriate diagnosis given their experiences (Herlihy & Corey, 2013).

Gender-sensitive psychotherapy also requires an intentionally established and maintained egalitarian relationship between clients and the therapist throughout the therapy process. The psychotherapist should consciously share power and responsibility with the client while recognizing and continuously admitting that there is inherently an imbalance of power. It is essential to be open in receiving feedback and demystifying the therapeutic process to minimize the inherent power differential and build trust. The psychotherapist must avoid acting as the "expert" and providing guidance and opinion (Herlihy & Corey, 2013). As an alternative, a healthy alliance is crucial at each stage of the therapeutic process, including conceptualization, goal setting, treatment planning, and the termination process. Psychotherapists should be fully trained as gender-sensitive therapists. They must be able to discuss clients' experiences with gender and oppression to normalize their experiences and contribute to promoting an egalitarian relationship. Gender-sensitive psychotherapists strive to be continuously reflective and mindful of not imposing their own principles and standards. Instead, they create a safe environment for clients to carefully and securely delve into their own options and feel empowered to choose for themselves (Herlihy & Corey, 2013).

Traditional gender roles and family structure have been shown to affect both men and women in families adversely. As psychotherapists, we generally expect that the process of therapy can be very influential in changing the vicious cycle for men to be distant and for women to be central in their families' lives. More specifically, gender-sensitive psychotherapists generally seek ways to fully engage men and hold them equally responsible for any change in the relational dynamics with women in the context of family therapy. Yet, in a very thought-provoking study in the US by Wheeler (1985), two seemingly contradictory issues were simultaneously endorsed. Psychotherapists claimed that it is very important for them to avoid placing all the primary responsibility for change in the family on women. However, almost all of the interventions identified focused on influencing and pressuring women to change, while few interventions were directed and pressured men to change. The central and significant body of literature in the US covering the topic of women in psychotherapy reveals that some therapists are conscious of how they are treating women differently (Goodrich *et al.*, 1988; Goodrich, 1991; Walters *et al.*, 1991). However, even though feminist family therapy has evolved toward an integrated model of gender sensitivity, it often lacks explicit ideas and suggestions on how therapists should engage men in the family change in more fundamental ways.

In their initial evaluations of family therapy, Goldner (1985) and Hare-Mustin and Marecek (1988) discussed that the therapist often perceives men as less competent than women in negotiating the therapeutic relationship. Thus, men's perceived helplessness and vulnerability in the therapy room provide the therapist an implicit yet powerful message of "if I am not protected here, I'm not coming back" (Goldner, 1985: 40). These writers believe that, historically, this inherent expectation and the accompanying and entrenched power and control dynamic forces the therapist to carefully choose interventions to appeal to his position in the family. On the other hand, psychotherapists have to be careful not to blame men when they have difficulties engaging male clients. These perspectives are very constrictive in our work with men in families.

Male socialization to act masculine creates expectations for men to be strong, super competent, rational, and analytical in the way they express themselves, which is not the typical way we expect clients to express themselves in the therapy room. When masculinity is highly valued in Western cultures, these kinds of behavior make men appear vulnerable and may even reveal character weakness. Further, the rigid definition of masculinity socializes men to believe that self-reflection and soul-searching will lead to humiliation and rejection. As psychotherapists, we often see men who seek help being pressured by family, work, or the court system to attend therapy and are unwilling participants. Those who decide to start treatment without others' pressure may want to be vulnerable, but they still struggle with being loyal to their masculine mystique. Further, therapists may, unconsciously and unintentionally, view men who seek therapy in more negative terms based on their own cultural ideologies of masculinity (Dienhart, 2001).

Gender and Supervision

A psychotherapist's professional development highly depends on a healthy and balanced supervisory relationship. When it comes to gender-sensitive supervision, supervisors must be able to use the relationship as an opportunity to support, educate, challenge, and model. This means that the supervisor has to develop and show a special level of awareness of self and society. It is absolutely crucial to challenge our own biases, prejudices, and gender-related stereotypes. Gender sensitivity is one of our most compelling and evocative attributes and

often is one of the most sensitive and delicate areas of our personal exploration. Its sensitive nature makes it imperative that the entire supervision process
happens with a high level of sensitivity to gender and contextual issues within
the most explicit ethical boundaries. These boundaries provide a safe environment for the personal growth of the supervisee, while also modeling gender-
sensitive professional behavior for the next generation of psychotherapists.

Conclusion

Based on the review of theories and research studies, we can explain what it
means to be male, female, and rarely a nonbinary person in societies. The most
fundamental perspective about gender differences focuses on the unequal distribution of power, socialization, and inherent differences between men, women,
and nonbinary individuals. In the US, for example, men as a group (read White
men) have more economic, political, social, and physical (all men) power than
most women. However, males and females are socialized to become different
beings as well. They receive strong messages from family, school, and media
that continue to be heavily overloaded with sex-role messages representing very
different sets of acceptable behaviors for boys and girls.

These strict but unconscious social rules and expectations create extraordinarily contrasting psychological environments for development based on gender.
As for inherent differences, those attributes stereotypically identified women's
traits historically had been dismissed as having little value. Specifically, within
the field of psychology, the model of the healthy adult has traditionally and
even today been described through masculine characteristics. This rigid societal
context creates distinct power differentials for men, women, and nonbinaries,
reinforcing expectations and actions. Gender is a significant social variable,
and its impact should be apparent in psychotherapy and supervision. These
parallel processes need to be continuously examined within the larger context
of society. Finally, the minimization of within-group experience while exagger-
ating between-group experiences seriously reduces the potential for individual
difference. Additionally, we should never forget that even though much of our
understanding about gender differences has been brought up and discussed by
women and as part of their movement, gender stereotyping has the potential
for bias and discrimination that affect both men and women.

References

Afifi, M. (2007). Gender differences in mental health. *Singapore Medical Journal, 48*(5),
385–391.
Ashraf, F. (2018). Social Construction of Masculinity and Femininity. *Gender and Inclusive
Perspective in Education.* Delhi: AkiNik Publications, 67–82.
Coltrane, S., & Adams, M. (2008). *Gender and Families* (Vol. 5). Lanham, MD: Rowman
& Littlefield.
Deleuze, G., & Guattari, F. (1983). *Anti-Oedipus: Capitalism and Schizophrenia.* Trans. Robert
Hurley, Mark Seem and Helen R. Lane. Minneapolis: University of Minnesota Press.

Deleuze, G., & Guattari, F. (1987). A *Thousand Plateaus: Capitalism and Schizophrenia*. Trans. Brian Massumi. Minneapolis: University of Minnesota Press.

Dienhart, A. (2001). Engaging men in family therapy: Does the gender of the therapist make a difference? *Journal of Family Therapy, 23*(1), 21–45.

Goldner, V. (1985). Feminism and Family Therapy. https://doi.org/10.1111/j.1545-5300.1985.00031.x.

Goodrich, T. J. (1991) Women, power, and family therapy, *Journal of Feminist Family Therapy, 3*:1-2, 5–37, DOI: 10.1300/J086v03n01_02

Goodrich, T. J., Rampage, C., Ellman, B., & Halstead, K. (1988) *Feminist Family Therapy: A Casebook*. New York: W. W. Norton.

Haig, D. (2004). The inexorable rise of gender and the decline of sex: Social change in academic titles, 1945–2001. *Archives of Sexual Behaviour, 33*(2), 87–96.

Haralambos, M., & Holborn, M. (2014). Sex and Gender: Culture, Socialization and Identity. *Sociology: Themes and Perspectives*, 8th edn. London: HarperCollins.

Hare-Mustin, R. T., & Marecek, J. (1988). The meaning of difference: Gender theory, postmodernism, and psychology. *American Psychologist, 43*(6), 455–464. https://doi.org/10.1037/0003-066X.43.6.455

Herlihy, B., & Corey, G. (2013). Feminist therapy. In G. Corey (Ed.), *Theory and Practice of Counseling and Psychotherapy* (9th ed., pp. 360–394). Belmont, CA: Brooks/Cole, Cengage Learning.

Irigaray, L. (1984). *An Ethics of Sexual Difference*. Trans. Carolyn Burke and Gillian Gill. Ithaca, NY: Cornell University Press.

Irigaray, L. (1985a). *Speculum of the Other Woman*. Trans. Gillian Gill. Ithaca, NY: Cornell University Press.

Irigaray, L. (1985b). *This Sex Which is Not One*. Trans. Catherine Porter with Carolyn Burke. Ithaca, NY: Cornell University Press.

Irigaray, L. (2008). *Conversations*. London: Bloomsbury Publishing.

Jablonka, E., & Lamb, M. J. (2005). *Evolution in Four Dimensions: Genetic, Epigenetic, Behavioral, and Symbolic Variation in the History of Life*. Cambridge, MA: MIT Press.

Kendall, D. (2003). *Sociology in Our Time*. Belmont, CA: Wadsworth/Thomas Learning.

Kerr, B., & Godfrey-Smith, P. (2002). Individualist and multi-level perspectives on selectionin structured populations. *Biology & Philosophy, 17*, 477–517. https://doi.org/10.1023/a:1020504900646

Lindqvist, A., Sendén, M. G., & Renström, E. A. (2021). What is gender, anyway: a review of the options for operationalising gender. *Psychology & Sexuality, 12*(4), 332–344.

Lorber, J. (1994). *Paradoxes of Gender*. New Haven, CT: Yale University Press.

Mahtab, N. (2015). *Women, Gender and Development: Contemporary Issues*. AH Development Publishing House.

Mcleod, S. (2004). *Cognitive Dissonance*. Retrieved from https://www.simplypschology.org,

Meyerowitz, J. (2008). A history of "gender." *The American Historical Review, 113*(5), 1346–1356.

Oakley, A. (1974). *The Sociology of Housework*. Oxford: Martin Robertson.

Obi, E. A. (2018). Understanding the theories of gender. In E. A. Obi, C. A. Obiora, N. Ebisi & I. E. Ezeabasili (Eds), *Contemporary Gender Issues*. Onitsha, Nigeria: AbbotCommunication Ltd.

Okasha, S. (2006). *Evolution and the Levels of Selection*. Oxford/New York: Clarendon Press; Oxford University Press.

Schaefer, R. T. (2005). *Sociology* (9th ed.). Boston: McGraw Hill.

Scobey-Thal, J. (2014). Third Gender: A Short History, Foreign Policy. https://foreig npolicy.com/2014/06/30/third-gender-a-short-history/

Tomasello, M. (1999). *The Cultural Origins of Human Cognition*. Cambridge, MA/ London: Harvard University Press.

Tomasello, M., Carpenter, M., Call, J., Behne, T., & Moll, H. (2005). Understanding and sharing intentions: The origins of cultural cognition. *Behavioral and Brain Sciences*, *28*(5), 675–691.

UNESCO's Gender Mainstreaming Implementation Framework (2003). https://unes doc.unesco.org/ark:/48223/pf0000131854

Walby, S. (1990). *Theorizing Patriarchy*. Oxford: Basil Blackwell.

Walters, M., Carter, B., Papp, P., & Silverstein, O. (1991). *The Invisible Web: Gender Patterns in Family Relationships*. New York: Guilford Press.

Wheeler, F. D. (1985). The Theory and Practice of Feminist-Informed Family Therapy: A Delphie Study. Purdue University. ProQuest Dissertations Publishing, 8529347.

Wilson, D. S., & Wilson, E. O. (2007). Rethinking the theoretical foundation of sociobiology. *Quarterly Review of Biology*, *82*(4), 327–348.

2 Masculinity in Global Contexts

Introduction

The original Greek term 'patriarch' intended to include the essence of the logic of patriarchy as an absolutely linear legitimacy of power and meaning. The current internalized and globalized hegemonic forms of male order are the results of centuries of mythical, metaphysical, systematic, political, socioeconomic, legal, and linguistic advancement through a Eurocentric realm, spread through colonization, globalization, and development cross-culturally. Male order can be characterized as discriminating, regulating, and categorizing a set of nonrepresentational and binary perspectives focused on control, order, linear progress, expansion, and growth without accountability. It seems evident that the more men participate in patriarchy, the more they become disconnected from the experiences of others. Men who are socialized within a strict patriarchal societal structure are pressured to define themselves relative to what it means to be a man and how men are expected to behave. These pressures have been internalized and shaped men's attitudes and practices in relation to women. Even when men go against this grain, resist such forces, and seek to establish respectful and equal relationships with women, the expectations of patriarchal perspectives have been internalized within their psyches. Thus, if gender hierarchies were going to change in any society, it is imperative for men to understand and challenge the powerful influence of patriarchy.

Men and Masculinity

In *The Myth of Masculinity*, Joseph Pleck (1981) discusses the gender role strain paradigm as one of the leading perspectives in modern critical thinking about masculinity. This paradigm proposes that appropriate gender roles are determined by parents, teachers, and peers' prevailing gender ideology imposed on the developing child. The strain paradigm also states that contemporary gender roles are contradictory and inconsistent, and many individuals violate these gender roles, which has more negative consequences for men than women. Further, the traditional masculinity ideology is a multidimensional construct. It includes the male gender norms of avoiding all things feminine,

DOI: 10.4324/9781003088189-3

restricting one's emotional reactions, acting tough and aggressive, being auton-omous and self-reliant, attaining status at any costs, exhibiting non-relational attitudes toward sexuality, and showing hatred toward homosexuals.

Pleck (1995) discusses three categories of male gender role strains: discrep-ancy, dysfunction, and trauma. Discrepancy strain happens when men do not live up to their own internalized manhood ideal, based on traditional mascu-linity ideology. Dysfunction strain happens when men fulfill all requirements of the male behavioral and attitudinal code, even when they have negative consequences for themselves and for others who are close to them. Trauma strain happens from the tribulation of the male socialization process. In partic-ular, boys' emotional socialization process is highly suppressed and channeled against natural emotionality to the extent that adult males usually are less emo-tionally empathic than females. They are also more susceptible to expressing anger and frustration aggressively and transforming their vulnerable emotions like sadness, fear, and shame into anger. Thus, even though men have higher status and are privileged in our patriarchal societies relative to women, male socialization has long negatively affected women, men, children, and society.

Men and the Dilemma of Health

Boys' and men's health outcomes are considerably worse than girls' and women's globally (World Health Organization, 2014). However, this gendered inequality in health has not received national, regional, or global recognition or consideration from policymakers or healthcare providers. The fact that men's health tends to be worse than women's is now clear based on evidence from many sources worldwide. A research study done by the Institute for Health Metrics and Evaluation in 2010 by Wang and colleagues revealed that during the period from 1970 to 2010, women's life expectancy increased from 61.2 to 73.3 years, while male life expectancy increased from 56.4 to 67.5 years (Wang et al., 2012). Overall, by 2010, women were outliving men by an average of almost six years. According to the Global Health 2035 report, published in *The Lancet* in 2013, in countries classified as "least developed" by the United Nations, between 1992 and 2012, women's mortality rate fell faster than among men (Jamison et al., 2013). In the area with the lowest life expectancy at birth, such as central sub-Saharan Africa, on average, men were living 5.3 years less than women. This gap is even wider for men and women residing in Eastern Europe, where women in the Russian Federation lived longer than men by an average of 11.6 years.

Globally, men typically have easier access to better opportunities, privileges, and power than women, but their health outcomes are poorer. Based on studies done by the WHO, European Region's review of the social determinants of health, men's poorer survival rates are impacted by several factors. These include higher exposure to physical and chemical hazards, risk-taking behaviors, and lack of general help-seeking behaviors. Further, when men are ill, they are less likely to visit a doctor and, even when they seek medical advice, they are less likely to report on the symptoms of disease or illness (UCL Institute of Health Equity, 2013).

In 2010, 3.14 million men compared to 1.72 million women died from reasons associated with excessive alcohol use (Lim *et al.*, 2012). According to this study, excessive alcohol consumption for men is associated with masculinity traits. More importantly, in the GBD 2010 study, out of the 67 risk factors, 60 risk factors were related to more male than female deaths, and the top 10 risk factors were all more common in men (Lim *et al.*, 2012).

Furthermore, it seems as if globally, women tend to use health services more than men, even though this gap may reflect the fact that women use health services more during their reproductive years (Hawkes & Buse, 2013). Several studies in Africa reveal that these notions of masculinity highly increase the risk of infection with the human immunodeficiency virus (HIV) and prevent men from getting tested for HIV. They also have a hard time dealing with their HIV-positive status, following directives from nurses, and engaging in healthier behaviors (Baker *et al.*, 2014).

Lastly, the type of work men tend to perform in all societies is highly gendered and exposes men to occupations with higher morbidity and mortality rates. For example, in 2010, about 750,000 men died from occupationally related causes instead of just over 102,000 women (Lim *et al.*, 2012). A study conducted in Europe reported that 95 percent of all lethal accidents and 76 percent of all non-lethal accidents at work are experienced by men (Baker *et al.*, 2014). In the US, occupations like mining, agriculture, and fishing hire more men than women and have the highest risk of fatal occupational injury.

In most parts of the world, men are more likely to ignore and underreport being abused (Drijber *et al.*, 2013). They are also more prone to commit suicide (Ministry of Health, 2017; United Health Foundation, 2019). Men also have a propensity to have lower educational achievement than women (Ministry of Education, 2020), higher rates of incarceration (Ministry of Health, 2017), and higher rates of homelessness (Demographic Data Project, 2018; Hughes, 2021). However, these gender-based inequalities have received little national, regional, or global acknowledgment or attention from policymakers or providers, especially in healthcare (Baker *et al.*, 2014).

There seem to be several reasons causing these systemic health-based differences seen between men and women. Specific biological differences are linked to a gene, hormone's reproductive structure, and metabolism. They're also socially constructed issues like having lower social support, experiencing more significant levels of shame and stigma associated with support-seeking behaviors, and being less likely to report the symptoms and more likely to minimize symptoms of their disease or illness (Harvard Health, 2019).

Other factors contributing to these health-related differences are lower socioeconomic status, lower education level, and employment type. An affiliation with minority ethnics and sexual groups may also intensify men's morbidity and mortality rate compared to women, causing a lower quality of life (White *et al.*, 2020). Men also overly represent substance abusers, the homeless, family and interpersonal violence perpetrators, absent fathers and fathers separated from their children, sex addicts, and sex offenders, and victims of homicide, suicide, fatal automobile accidents, and lifestyle and stress-related catastrophic incidents.

Masculinity Identity Crisis

Anthropologists have revealed that different cultures universally construct a model of proper manhood that is typically challenging for men to achieve and, once achieved, can be very unstable (Gilmore, 1990). More importantly, men are more often under tremendous pressure to prove their masculinity than women are to prove their femininity (Ducat, 2004; Kimmel, 1996). Further, people can easily imagine how a man might lose his manhood if he cannot support a family or loses a job. Still, it is more complicated to describe a woman losing her womanhood (Vandello *et al.*, 2008). In other words, the ideal masculinity is challenging for men to achieve (O'Neil & Nadeau, 1999). They often have to engage in behaviors such as suppressing emotions and acting hyper-heterosexual to hold on to their masculinity.

One of the main areas where masculinity gets enacted and proven is the workplace, economic achievements, and high organizational status (Collinson & Hearn, 2005). Many ethnographic studies have examined how men's masculinity can be threatened at work and how men attempt to reaffirm their sense of power and masculinity. One great example is that men's masculinity is questioned when men work in highly feminized occupations, such as nurses or preschool teachers. Thus, men in these professions tend to use specific tactics to maintain their identity as men (Henson & Rogers, 2001). In contrast, when women work in highly masculine jobs, they are not socialized to use similar strategies to reaffirm their "true" femininity. Thus, work roles are the primary source of evaluating men's masculinity but not as central for assessing women's femininity, and men in these roles lose more status than women.

Cross-Cultural Gender Practices

Men's attitudinal support for or opposition to gender role equality is complex. Cross-culturally men may respect women in their personal lives but appreciate the broader power arrangements in their society that support men (Fleming *et al.*, 2013). Most men are in support of the patriarchal gender order. Their sympathy for gender equality issues is restricted, maybe even insincere, and is activated more concerning women in their own lives. While many men very much embrace the idea that women should have equal access to education and employment, only a small group of men practice gender equality in their attitude toward women as a whole. A much smaller group of men will intervene when other men behave in sexist or violent ways. Thus, men's behavior toward women related to them is protective while simultaneously preserving their own masculine societal benefit by not advocating for the same rights for all women.

Additionally, men's positions toward gender equality differ based on other forms of societal differences and inequalities, including race and ethnicity, education, and region. This makes sense since men's involvement in gender role issues is shaped by the gender relations of their local contexts and communities. Globally, some communities are characterized by more vigorous advocacy for gender equality, while others are characterized by traditional gender norms of male dominance and female subordination. Even in a single community or context, there is multiplicity in how men's peer cultures and groups impact their perception of women and issues related to equality (Flood, 2011, 2015; Flood & Russell, 2017). Globally, education has a meaningful but not exclusive impact on attitudes toward gender. The IMAGES surveys in eight countries showed positive associations between the level of education in the country and support for gender equality in six of these countries, but not for Brazil and India (Fleming *et al.*, 2013). Overall, these findings reveal that men's attitudes toward gender roles differ by the economic situation, family context, socialization experience, religious and political ideologies, race/ethnicity, and regional and historical contexts (Flood & Russell, 2017).

White Men and "The Other" Men Status

There seems to be a crisis when it comes to men's identity and masculinity due to the collapse of the idea that men define themselves by having a "good provider" role, which results in gender role strain. There seems to be a much bigger identity crisis for White, middle-class men who are no longer the "good providers" for their families compared to their fathers and their own expectations of themselves. Given that more women are now part of the workforce, White men are no longer the only provider. The Families and Work Institute (1995) stated that 55 percent of employed married women provide half or more of the household income.

The good-provider role is used to define masculinity in a significant way, so some White men are actively trying to create a new meaning for masculinity to balance work with family life, while others are in denial. In many instances, wives work full-time, but husbands still consider themselves their family's provider. They try to justify and rationalize that they make more money than their wives, or perhaps have a higher potential to earn more money, and are more committed to providing for the family compared to their wives. Other White men are gravitating toward organizations like the Promise Keepers (promisekeepers.org) and the Fatherhood Initiative (Horn & Blankenhorn, 1999) to try to return men to their "rightful place" as the "leader of his family" and dismiss the achievements of the women's movement.

It seems like men are trapped in a confusing situation caught between having greater power on the one hand and being vulnerable on the other hand. Furthermore, they do not have the incentives or psychological skills to process and understand the loss of the good-provider role. They collaboratively and reasonably resolve these issues with the women in their lives because of the power and the sense of entitlements they have accumulated in a patriarchal society. If they want to address any of these issues, they must learn how to process emotions against the male gender role socialization process.

The severe forms of gender role strain have long impacted men of color, gay or bisexual men, differently-abled men, and the lower socioeconomic class (women of color, conversely, always had to always work for the sake of economic necessity). This masculinity identity crisis may have intensified the ongoing role strain experienced by marginalized men in these groups. However, White middle- to upper-middle-class heterosexual men who were somewhat more protected from gender role strain have been impacted the most. It makes sense to assume that the masculinity identity crisis can potentially reduce the barriers between men who have been impacted by racism, classism, heterosexism, giving White, middle-class men more opportunities to have compassion and sympathize with the diverse groups of men. Further, the inconveniences of dominance in a patriarchal society should create an understanding among men of all classes, ethnic, and racial backgrounds. However, mainly because of the strange nature of the masculine identity crisis, in which gender remains invisible and does not get identified as the main source of gender role strain, not only do White men not sympathize with "the other" men, but they may also even perpetuate the strain.

Barriers to Achieving Gender Equality

There are many barriers to achieving gender equality, such as male peer pressure, societal customs and norms, and institutional policies like basing on-site childcare facilities on the number of female employees only, which influence gender-specific stereotypes (Brescoll *et al.,* 2012). These challenges, evident in various situations in all aspects of life, can be addressed through specific interventions to reduce gender inequality. Cross-culturally, men's power and authority are warranted based on religion, biology, cultural tradition, or organizational mission. Thus, men continue to benefit from these patriarchal dividends, and strong resistance to gender equality among certain men continues the systemic resistance to change. We have more awareness about the role of men in violence against women and sexual/reproductive health. However, gender socialization in the family, at school, and in the workplace are the underlying causes of these issues and reinforce gender stereotypes and assign expected gender roles.

In recent years, cross-culturally, men have been approached for three types of interventions: outreach, partnership, and gender transformation. In developed countries where the income is higher, like Australia, the United States, and Western European countries, outreach efforts have generally been aimed at men in bars, clubs, barbershops, sports clubs, schools, and the workplace. It has concentrated on helping men with weight loss, smoking cessation, and other lifestyle changes. The second method has focused on partnering with men to improve the health of women and children. For example, in Ghana, child vaccination programs that were designed to involve fathers more than mothers in decision-making about their children's use of preventive health services increased timely immunization (Baker *et al.*, 2014). Comparably, systematic examinations of studies done in developing countries have shown that engaging male partners in reproductive and sexual health decisions, including family planning, is highly beneficial (Baker *et al.*, 2014). A third method is to support interventions intended at gender transformation to reform gender roles leading to more equitable relationships between women and men. These interventions enhance protective sexual behaviors, counteract intimate partner violence, restrict discriminatory mindsets associated with gender, and reduce sexually transmitted diseases (Jamison *et al.*, 2013).

Further, these approaches may provide men better means for rebuilding the traditional male code in order to resolve the masculinity crisis and deal with their continuous predicament when it comes to connection and increasing healthier gender relations. Through the process of awareness, education, and support, men can overcome the emotional constraints that have been their legacy. It is helpful for men to realize that ideas widely shared among them and are mainly outside of their conscious awareness put them in a situation with a never-ending series of challenges. These challenges are often incompatible with their natural inclinations but oddly help them with the transient status of "manhood" imposed on them by their socialization patterns. Men must also realize that the feelings of shame they hold in their hearts about their perceived lack of masculinity are practically universal. There are always some very unpleasant costs connected with carrying the burdens of domination. Equality in gender relations can be attained when men are willing and guided to take these steps.

The Healing Power of Psychotherapy

As discussed in this chapter, regardless of how manhood has been defined and how men have been in dominant positions globally, many men experience pain and suffering based on socially constructed gender stereotypes and gain from a gender-equal society. These gender norms create pressure for men to be tough and the protectors and providers in often harsh environments. They may suffer from injuries, violence, crimes, imprisonments, and military service.

Men suffer from many forms of personal and institutional violence, primarily by other men, and can gain a great deal by advocating for gender equality in order to reduce violence against themselves. Moreover, challenging homophobia and other forms of discrimination against men due to their sexual orientation will certainly positively promote gender equality for heterosexual men and women. This is important since an oppressive 'status quo' is opposed and contested in both cases. Men also have been socialized not to deal with a whole range of emotions and experiences that are immensely rewarding and socially valued based on gender roles' strains. For example, in most cultures, men do not raise children, take care of their sick parents, or show affection and express their vulnerabilities when they are stressed out. It is very important to note that moving toward gender equality is not about promoting the loss of masculinity. It is about men as a group sharing and enjoying being part of a broader, healthier, safer, and richer cultural experience.

Psychotherapy can be beneficial to men because males' emotional reactions, vulnerability, and sensitivity are different from those of women. We habitually encourage men to be vulnerable, sensitive, or emotional the same way as women. However, internally this is not a comfortable process for men. The lack of an adequate role model prevents them from recapturing these qualities. At the same time, we should ask women to have the courage to access their power, take a stand, and put themselves before the relationship, not by imitating men but by following their own internalized process.

Most men come to see a therapist not because they want to change and think therapy can transform them but because they are in trouble with women in their lives. They have been asked to be more considerate and share feelings, and they want to accomplish this goal to stay connected to their spouses. However, outside of trying to please their partners, they don't know why they should learn to work on their emotional responses in their relationships. Other than trying to experience intimacy via sex, it is harder for them to experience intimate connections as inherently positive and pleasurable. Many men feel empowered and pleased when they can make their partners happy by providing for them, helping them, pleasuring them sexually, or making them feel physically safe. Cross-culturally, most men are raised by women, and if they have a positive relationship with their mothers, they want to make their partners happy just like they wanted to make their mothers happy. Thus, they are constantly looking for clues from their partners to assess how they are doing. If their partner is happy, they think everything is going well, and if she is not, they often think they need to fix the situation for their wife and rarely themselves. Further, based on how men have been socialized, they strive for a feeling of respect before reaching out to feel love. Thus, the most important task for men is to financially provide for their families, putting a massive amount of pressure on them. When they cannot adequately provide for their family, they struggle with feeling inadequate and anxious.

When there are power struggles in heterosexual relationships, it is helpful to ask men to shoulder the heavy burden of the relationship, do the heavy lifting, and take one for the team. Men often take on these responsibilities more easily since it has been part of their socialization, and women are often extremely grateful to them for doing it. Men act like men because they strive to be true to themselves based on how they have been socialized. If we want men to start a new journey to discover other aspects of themselves, they need women to partner with them and walk alongside them to help with this new journey. Finally, a man disconnected from his inner world is not attractive and not very easy to live with. We need to show men how to connect with their world, and that connecting helps them deal with the outer world much more easily.

Psychotherapists need to be specifically attuned that gender inequalities impact all aspects of family relationships and can be the operational base for workplace relational dynamics. At work, this can be officially through guidelines, strategies, and decision-making practices such as blocking promotion to those who work part-time, knowing that women may have to work part-time more often than men. It can also be through unofficial norms and standards such as decisions about including or excluding women in particular social and professional networks and using language to stereotype women.

Psychotherapists need to discuss how men benefit directly from gender equality at home and the workplace for many reasons. First, when the women and girls' family members are safe and treated fairly, men often feel better about themselves. Men's health and well-being are enhanced when limited definitions of masculinity are eased. Further, when women are promoters of relationship equality, men experience much greater stability and sexual satisfaction and have a higher level of involvement in their children's lives. Even at work, if all talents are honored and appreciated without a gender hierarchy, men can become more productive, creative, and use their diverse skills to become more successful.

Gay Men Relational Issues

Gay men's relationships sustain and thrive if there is a decent level of satisfaction for each partner. Psychotherapists must realize that even though gay men have been socialized as men, they must be mindful of not relying on unfair assumptions, stereotypes, or even prejudices when working with gay men. In the following section, some of the specific challenges for gay men that psychotherapists must be mindful of will be discussed.

Financial issues – gay male couples often can have some serious conflict around money. Based on their socialization, gay male couples compete with each other on physical appearance, social influence, and income. When financial issues happen in gay male relationships, it is related to the idea that men are still expected to be the "breadwinners cross-culturally." White men, particularly men with middle to higher socioeconomic status, are socialized to enjoy social privileges and receive more advantages without even asking for them. Gay men of color, on the other hand, face multiple challenges in managing social responses and burdens from being gay, a person of color, and gender role expectations. For example, heterosexual men still must deal with a lot of social pressure to earn more than their wives, and when heterosexual men earn less than their wives, they may feel shamed, envious, or disappointed. So, issues of each partner competing to be the breadwinner often arise in same-sex relationships for gay men. It is also explicit as well as implicit power dynamics for gay men that may create complexities needing relational therapy. In multicultural relationships, cultural differences can also add another source of challenge to the relationship. These cultural differences can relate to language, food, spirituality, traditions, habits, and money. Sometimes, conflictual issues related to money might be differences in culture, even the family culture, when both partners are of the same nationality/ethnicity. Couples therapy should engage the gay couple to discuss gender dynamics and male socialization, helping the partners understand that a healthy relationship should involve fewer battles about who makes more money or dominates the relationship. More accurately, it's about helping them understand that they have a partnership where both partners are stakeholders in the relationship. However, since men are generally taught to control and dominate from childhood, honoring this equal partnership and not competing about money is very hard for them.

Furthermore, heterosexual couples up until recently were the only group that had the legal recognition of their relationships. Gay men were two unrelated individuals under one roof, especially for legal and tax purposes. They are socialized to think independently, and mixing two individual incomes is mentally and emotionally challenging and only softens with increased time and trust. Besides this, heterosexual couples are socialized to combine their incomes more readily. For generations, they see their parents model this division in financial responsibilities by having joint bank accounts, filing for taxes jointly, and accessing survivor benefits. Couples therapy should include discussions to brainstorm, identify, evaluate, and implement specific money management strategies to help both partners make equal contributions based on their income, even if they have different earning potentials.

Sexuality and sexual relationship – gay male couples are much more likely to contemplate or even decide not to be in an exclusive sexual relationship with a cultural and historical root. Some aspects of this choice are the men's socialization regarding sexual behavior. In general, the idea of another man having sex with their partner/spouse may be appealing for gay men. Generally, men, particularly gay men, may have a greater capacity for casual sex without much foreplay and separating sex from love. Thus, when it comes to sexuality, gay couples' relationships are very different from heterosexual relationships, so psychotherapists should not use the information and experiences they have about heterosexual couples' sex life with a gay male couple's sex life. The dynamics are vastly different and don't translate culturally, physically, socially, or emotionally. Gay men need to be counseled to understand these differences and not directly compare them to heterosexual relationships. Psychotherapists must validate their experiences and allow gay male couples to discuss their sexuality separate from heteronormative expectations and also independent of even other gay male relationships. Topics related to monogamy, frequency, type of sex, BDSM, and even time management discussions are very different and must be discussed openly.

Housework – the equal contribution to household chores is a typical topic of conversation in couple therapy. While couples expect to divide the list of everyday household chores fairly, women are still doing most of the household chores associated with cleaning, organizing, and monitoring household tasks. Overall, men are still socialized to concentrate on being the provider and working outside the home or doing more physical/mechanical duties like cleaning and maintaining cars or working in their backyard. So, when heterosexual couples sustain a fairer division of household labor at home, they define themselves as nontraditional, behaving outside of these ingrained social expectations. For gay male couples, these domestic components can create tension about who does what and is expected to do what. There are no traditional gender roles to point everyone in the right direction, and there are no role models. In couples therapy in general, we have couples list all the household chores as exhaustively and comprehensively as possible. Based on a mix of skills, desires, and expectations, they decide who does what, and of course, the primary key is flexibility with these rules and expectations. The tricky part is when one partner has a very demanding job with many hours outside the house, and one partner has many more hours at home and can decide what it means to contribute equally. The crucial part of the discussion in therapy is often what feels fair, where both partners are expected to be making a very subjective equal contribution to the relationship. So, the challenge is trying to achieve a sense of fairness without one partner feeling forced to do too many domestic tasks, which by itself is outside of masculine identity norms and associated historically with women's tasks, which somehow have less value. In psychotherapy with gay male couples, psychotherapists must identify and process issues related to sexism and how family-of-origin modeling can create this duality in performing tasks that can create tension in the relationship.

Children – it has only recently been that gay male couples have had relatively adequate social support for having kids, either through fostering, adoption, or surrogacy. Men generally need more support when raising children by themselves, and gay men are no exception. However, one important distinction between heterosexual and gay male couples is that men in heterosexual relationships are expected to have children with pressure from parents, siblings, and peers. Still, gay male couples are expected not to have children. Gay men cannot experience accidental pregnancy either. Thus, they have to be very intentional about having a child without having any role models or knowing how to raise a child without relying on societal expectations of gender norms. For gay fathers, there are no gender stereotypes to lead the way in helping them make parenting boys and girls work. Psychotherapy sessions can be beneficial in creating a safe environment for gay male parents to process their insecurities and make parenting work.

Family – family dynamics are always complex, but for gay male relationships, it has been even more complicated. For example, caring for an aging parent is similar for heterosexual and gay male couples. Also, in family relationships with the in-laws, there may be some hostility for all kinds of reasons related to ethnicity, religion, socioeconomic status, or nationality that may create some tension in the couple's relationship. The risks are higher for gay male relationships because at least one homophobic person seems to be in every family. This puts gay men in an awkward position to confront any explicit or implicit hostile behavior toward their partner, which creates an extra burden on gay men's male relationships. In psychotherapy, family member conflicts can be attended through role-plays, role reversal/rehearsal, and family therapy.

Politics – gay male couples are more impacted by political issues related to laws and other societal changes than heterosexual couples. There are many debates about gay couples' legal and social status changes, and heterosexual couples are not affected. All states in the US and countries that legally accept marriage equality are impacting gay couples positively. In contrast, states and countries vehemently against gay marriage try to de-legitimize same-sex marriages, often based on religion, which affects gay couples negatively. This creates an extra layer of stress on the relationship. Gay male couples do better relationally and socially when they identify with other same-sex or straight couples who can provide support.

Additionally, due to all these challenges, gay male couples tend to be more politically conscious and active by joining protests, writing letters, attending campaigns, observing boycotts, or making donations compared to heterosexual couples. This is because their rights and sometimes existence are challenged, which puts more stress on the relationships. Psychotherapy should acknowledge the existence of these challenges and validate their feelings as well as help gay couples find ways to find a supportive group to share their pain. Psychotherapists can also advocate for social justice, write to political figures, and do presentations and advocacy work on behalf of this group. In summary, psychotherapists have to bear in mind that there are all kinds of stressors on gay male relationships, from dating and sexual orientation to all the political, religious, and cultural wars, nationally and globally. Thus, our job is to understand these challenges and help gay male couples experience better quality relationships.

Conclusion

Cross-culturally, there is a systemic pattern of ideological and concrete practices in which power relations between men and women are continuously and consistently created and recreated as meaningful. This gender order in any given society forms the way masculinities and femininities are understood and organized. Every known society distinguishes between women and men, even though there are differences in how these distinctions are drawn. However, the hierarchical ordering of these relationships defines men, and men's relationships are not necessary. For example, the economic order is a systematic ordering of people's relationship to production and consumption, creating the same gender order in the capitalist, feudal, or communist context.

It may seem strange, but gender order does not have to be patriarchal. It could also be egalitarian or even matriarchal. Suppose we use the concept of gender order instead of the idea of patriarchy. In that case, we can argue against tendencies to this universalist idea that the existence of patriarchy should not be assumed for each specific society. Thus, instead of portraying women and men as puppets of a patriarchal system, we should acknowledge the active part all individuals play in the creation and recreation of gender relationships, which can open doors for the possibility of social change. The gender order and specific nature of gendered relationships should be a dynamic process formed by societal demands and transformed. It can be shaped by the activities and desires of individuals who are themselves formed as part of these interactions. The femininity and masculinity that are formed and created by these counterbalancing forces will never be static but dynamic and, more often than not, always inconsistent and even contradictory.

White *et al.* (2011) have discussed that public and policy action to improve men's health should aim first at schools because this is where they learn most of the stereotypes about masculinity. These public and policy actions should promote men's health and well-being in the workplace. The other critical area for policy change is providing health services for marginalized men from different minority groups, men in the prison system, and gay men, all of whom have a higher incumbrance with disease and early death than other men.

In summary, the best way to address these issues men face is to pay closer attention to shame and stigma in accessing support services, especially in the healthcare system. It is utterly essential to reduce men's risk-taking and gender norm-based behaviors through psychotherapeutic work. This work can nurture more significant self-examination, self-awareness, emotional and social awareness, expression, emotional regulation skills, communication, and interpersonal skills and provide the emotional support they need and deserve.

References

Baker, P., Dworkin, S. L., Tong, S., Banks, I., Shand, T., & Yamey, G. (2014). The men's health gap: men must be included in the global health equity agenda. *Bulletin of the World Health Organization, 92,* 618–620. doi: http://dx.doi.org/10.2471/BLT.13.132795

Brescoll., V. L. Uhlmann., E. L., Moss-Racusin, C., & Sarnell, L. (2012). Masculinity, status, and subordination: Why working for a gender stereotype violator causes men to lose status. *Journal of Experimental Social Psychology, 48(1),*354–357.

Collinson, D. L., & Hearn, J. (2005). Men and masculinities in work, organizations and management. In M. Kimmel, J. Hearn, & R. W. Connell (Eds), *Handbook of Studies on Men and Masculinities* (pp. 289–310). Thousand Oaks, CA and London: Sage Publications.

Demographic Data Project. (2018). *Data Visualization: Gender and Individual Homelessness.* National Alliance to End Homelessness. https://endhomelessness.org/resource/data-visualization-gender-disparities-inhomelessness/

Drijber, B. C., Reijnders, U. J., & Ceelen, M. (2013). Male victims of domestic violence. *Journal of Family Violence, 28(2),* 173–178. https://link.springer.com/article/10.1007/s10896-012-9482-9

Ducat, S. J. (2004). *The Wimp Factor: Gender Gaps, Holy wars, and the Politics of Anxious Masculinity.* Boston, MA: Beacon Press.

Families and Work Institute. (1995). *Women: The New Providers.* Benton Harbor, MI: The Whirlpool Foundation.

Fleming, P. J., Barker, G., McCleary-Sills, J., & Morton, M. (2013). *Engaging Men and Boys in Advancing Women's Agency: Where We Stand and New Directions.* Gender Equality & Development. Washington, DC: World Bank.

Flood, M. (2011). Involving men in efforts to end violence against women. *Men and Masculinities, 14*(3), 358–377.

Flood, M. (2015). Work with men to end violence against women: A critical stocktake. *Culture, Health & Sexuality, 17* (supp. 2), 159–176.

Flood, M., & Russell, G.. (2017). *Men Make a Difference: How to Engage Men on Gender Equality.* Sydney: Diversity Council Australia.

Gilmore, D. D. (1990). *Manhood in the Making: Cultural Concepts of Masculinity.* New Haven, CT: Yale University Press.

Harvard Health (2019, August 26) *Mars vs. Venus: The gender gap in health-harvard health publishing.* Harvard Health (August 26). https://www.health.harvard.edu/newsletter_article/mars-vs-venus-the-gender-gap-in-health/

Hawkes, S., & Buse, K. (2013). Gender and global health: evidence, policy, and inconvenient truths. *The Lancet. 381*(9879):1783–1787.

Henson, K. D., & Rogers, J. K. (2001). "Why Marcia you've changed!" Male clerical temporary workers doing masculinity in a feminized occupation. *Gender & Society, 15*(2), 218–238.

Horn, W. F., & Blankenhorn, D. (1999). *The Fatherhood Movement: A Call to Action.* American Quarterly. https://www.fatherhood.gov/sites/default/files/resource_files/e000000395_0.pdf

Hughes, C. (2021, July 5). *New Zealand: Homeless population in Auckland by gender 2018.* Statista. https://www.statista.com/statistics/1029005/new-zealand-homeless-population-in-auckland-bygender/#:~:text=According%20to%20a%20survey%20on,as%20neither%20male%20nor%20female/

Jamison, D. T., Summers, L. H., Alleyne, G., Arrow, K. J., Berkley, S., Binagwaho, A., & Yamey, G. (2013). Global Health 2035: a world converging within a generation. *The Lancet, 382*(9908), 1898–1955.

Kimmel, M. (1996). *Manhood in America: A Cultural History.* New York: The Free Press.

Lim, S. S., Vos, T., Flaxman, A. D., Danaei, G., Shibuya, K., Adair-Rohani, H.,…& Pelizzari, P. M. (2012). A comparative risk assessment of burden of disease and injury attributable to 67 risk factors and risk factor clusters in 21 regions, 1990-2010: a systematic analysis for the Global Burden of Disease Study. *The Lancet, 380* (9859), 2224–2260.

Ministry of Education – Education Counts. School Leaver's Attainment. (2020). https://www.educationcounts.govt.nz/indicators/main/student-engagementparticipation/retention_of_students_in_senior_secondary_schools

Ministry of Health (2017). Data story overview https://www.health.govt.nz/system/files/documents/pages/data-story-overview-suicide-preventionstrategy-april2017newmap.pdf

O'Neil, J. M., & Nadeau, R. A. (1999). Men's gender-role conflict, defense mechanism, and self-protective defensive strategies: Explaining men's violence against women from a gender-role socialization perspective. In M. Harway & J. M. O'Neil (Eds.), *What Causes Men's Violence Against Women.* Thousand Oaks, CA: Sage Publications.

Pleck, J. H. (1981). *The Myth of Masculinity.* Cambridge, MA: MIT Press.

Pleck, J. H. (1995). The gender role strain paradigm: An update. In R. F. Levant & W. S. Pollack (Eds.), *A new Psychology of Men* (pp. 11–32). New York: Basic Books/Hachette Book Group.

UCL Institute of Health Equity. (2013). *Review of Social Determinants and the Health Divide in the WHO European Region: Final report.* Institiute of Health Equity. http://www.inst ituteofhealthequity.org/projects/who-european-review

United Health Foundation. (2019). *2019 Senior Report: Health Disparities by Gender.* United Health Foundation. https://www.americashealthrankings.org/learn/reports/2019-senior-report/findings-health-disparities-bygender

Vandello, J. A., Bosson, J. K., Cohen, D., Burnaford, R. M., & Weaver, J. R. (2008). Precarious manhood. *Journal of Personality and Social Psychology, 95*(6), 1325.

Wang, H., Dwyer-Lindgren, L., Lofgren, K. T., Rajaratnam, J. K., Marcus, J. R., & Levin-Rector, A. (2012). Age-specific and sex-specific mortality in 187 countries, 1970–2010: a systematic analysis for the Global Burden of Disease Study 2010. *The Lancet, 380*(9859), 2071–2094.

White, A., McKee, M., Richardson, N., isser, R., Madsen, S.A., Sousa, B. C., Hogston, R., Zatonski, W., & Makara, P. (2011). Europe's men need their own health strategy. *BMJ.* Nov 29;343:d7397. doi: 10.1136/bmj.d7397. PMID: 22127516.

White, J. J., Dangerfield, D. T., Donovan, E., Miller, D., & Grieb, S. M. (2020). Exploring the role of LGBT affirming churches in health promotion for Black sexual minority men. *Culture, Health & Sexuality, 22*(10), 1191–1206. http://dx.doi.org/10.1080/13691058.2019.1666429

World Health Organization. (2014). *Men's Health.* World Health Organization. http://www.euro.who.int/en/health-topics/health-determinants/gender/activities/mens-health

3 Women's Rights in
Global Contexts

Introduction

Women and girls are half of the globe's population as well as half of the world's potential. Gender equality as a fundamental human right is vital for healthy growth in all societies because it enhances full human potential and helps with sustainable development. Furthermore, empowering women stimulates productivity and economic growth. Sadly, complete equality of rights and opportunities between men and women in all cultures has not been achieved. It is imperative that societies cross-culturally stop many forms of gender violence and provide equal access to quality education, health, and economic resources. They must also allow equal involvement and partnership in political and social decision-making and leadership for men, women, boys, girls, and nonbinary individuals. Mr. António Guterres, the UN Secretary-General, states that we must achieve gender equality and empower women and girls and see this problem as the greatest human rights challenge in our world (UN, 2020).

Unfortunately, gender equality has not been fully achieved by any country internationally. Iceland, Norway, Finland, and Sweden take the lead in their advances toward closing the gender gap (Hausmann *et al.*, 2010) by creating a reasonably equal distribution of income, assets, and economic prospects for men and women. The most considerable gender inequalities are predominantly in the Middle East, Africa, and South Asia (Hausmann *et al.*, 2010). Interestingly enough, some countries in the same region, like Lesotho, South Africa, and Sri Lanka, outrank the United States in gender equality (Hausmann *et al.*, 2010). The following section is devoted to the issues girls and women face globally, especially in developing countries. It is essential to mention that the status of women in many of these countries is part of more significant contextual issues related to colonialism and extraction of raw resources by European colonists, which impacts both men and women. However, in this chapter, we concentrate on women's issues.

Women's Issues from an International Perspective

Overall, there are many vital issues affecting girls and women worldwide, such as access to education, prospects of employment, reproductive health, maternal

DOI: 10.4324/9781003088189-4

health, gender-based violence, child marriage, female genital mutilation, water and sanitation, and gender equality. Each one will be discussed briefly below to create a context for understanding human rights globally.

Access to education: According to a report by UNESCO in 2013, 31 million girls of primary school age were not attending school, and approximately one out of four girls in developing countries did not complete elementary school education, which means there are untapped girls' power resources. On the other hand, education is vital to better decision-making since educated women tend to get married later, have a lower rate of maternal and infant mortality, have resources to raise healthy kids, are able to find meaningful work, and earn more money.

Prospects of employment: The wage gap is a big problem for women gaining economic independence globally. The US is one of the wealthiest and best-developed countries on earth, but women encounter significant disparity as workers by earning on average only $0.77 for every $1 made by men. Globally, women earn on average one-tenth of the world's income even though their total work hours are two-thirds of all working hours (OECD, 2018). Enabling women to earn based on their fair contributions to the world economy would benefit all communities since women, compared to men, are likely to spend most of their money on their families and communities (OECD, 2018).

Reproductive health: In developing countries, there seem to be about 225 million women that do not have access to family planning. This appears to be contributing to 74 million unplanned pregnancies and 36 million abortions annually (Sedghe *et al.*, 2016). If societies educate women about reproductive health and allow them to be in charge of their own bodies and make reproductive health decisions, we can significantly decrease unsafe abortions and maternal deaths by 70 percent. This can help countries preserve valuable resources that are generally used for pregnancy-related costs.

Maternal health: The World Health Organization (2016, 2019) reports that approximately 800 women die every day from preventable causes related to complications with pregnancy, which equals about 300,000 lives per year. Regardless of constant improvements in medical treatment, rates of maternal mortality and morbidity and premature infant birth have been rising in the US. It should be alarming that maternal and infant mortality rates in the US are considerably greater than those in comparably large and prosperous countries, and minorities are at higher risk for inadequate maternal and infant health outcomes (Singh, 2010). Though issues related to maternal health are directly linked to racial/ethnic disparities across the US, there are also broader inequalities across specific states and rural communities cross-culturally (Singh & Stella, 2019).

Gender-based violence: The World Health Organization report (2013) states that one in three women encounter physical or sexual violence in their lifetimes, including domestic abuse like physical assault, rape, and sex trafficking. This gender-based violence prevents so many women from living happy, healthy, and fulfilling lives.

Child marriage: Becoming a child bride impacted an estimated 140 million girls between 2011 and 2020 (WHO, 2020). This creates multiple issues for girls who marry before age 18, including not continuing their education and being at risk for a complicated pregnancy and premature childbirth. They may also be more at risk for intimate partner violence.

Female Genital Mutilation: Female Genital Mutilation is characterized by WHO (2020, para. 5) as: "procedures that intentionally alter or cause injury to the female genital organs for non-medical reasons." This is a multifaceted and complicated issue intertwined with misusing and misunderstanding religion, which also adds cultural consequences for those who practice it. The widespread agreement among many in the international community is that female genital mutilation inflicts terrible health outcomes, infringes on a child's rights to be safe and not harmed, and fosters unfair inequality between men and women.

Water and sanitation: Access to clean drinking water is essential for girls and women since, in many developing countries, they are tasked with fetching and preserving water. This is a very time-consuming task and, at times, can be dangerous. Furthermore, girls and women have unique needs to access sanitary facilities during their menstrual cycles. In Africa, research shows that girls that do not have access to appropriate clean facilities do not attend schools during their menstrual periods for fear of embarrassment or stigma (UNICEF and WSSCC, 2005).

Gender equality: According to UN Women (2020), 95 percent of countries are run by a male head of state. Equality is a recurrent problem for women and girls regarding disproportionate access to education for girls in developing countries or disparity in pay in the workplace.

These issues seem so specific to girls and women. However, focusing on them will positively impact everyone around the globe. At the international level, we need to empower the voices of women. Currently, women and young girls in all places encounter enormous arrays of challenges, starting with their inability to access clean water, food, quality education, employment, and the real threat of gender-based violence. Girls' and women's perspectives and experiences must help us form our shared future. In the next section, the status of women in the US will be discussed to create specific frameworks for women's progress both globally and nationally.

Status of Women in the United States

We have witnessed lots of progress in the US for women regarding political participation. More women are serving in the House and Senate than ever before, and for the first time in history, the vice president is a woman. The following section discusses that women in the US still find gender equality tenuous and mostly not achievable despite these gains.

Women and power – One of the struggles behind work and family-related governmental policies is not allowing women to be involved in positions of power.

Women are not represented in the corporate boardrooms, courthouses, or political leadership positions. Women who do not hold senior positions in the US create significant issues, including getting paid at a lower rate and dealing with all kinds of discrimination. We need to understand that not allowing women to hold leadership roles prevents real advancement for all people and not just women.

Patriarchy – One of the significant challenges facing women in the US is patriarchy, especially in the political field. In the US, irrespective of a woman's experience, education, or aptitudes and capabilities, the patriarchal nature of US society promotes the idea that women are less competent and less capable than men. Patriarchy cleverly convinces people that powerful and smart women disturb the social order instead of being a fundamental part of the political and social system. The media coverage of women as political figures focuses on their fashions instead of their ideas on policy and their positions on social issues. It is no wonder that the US is so far behind the rest of the world in electing a woman as president. Muslim-dominated countries like Pakistan, Indonesia, Bangladesh, Turkey, Kosovo, and many others have had 13 women serving as either prime ministers or presidents since the early 1980s (Wills *et al.*, 2019). Furthermore, women have held the highest office of leadership in Liberia, India, the United Kingdom, Dominica, and many other nations across the globe, but the United States is still behind.

Educational opportunities – Regardless of many gains for women's equality, educational inequality has been one of the women's biggest challenges. The modern feminist movements have been challenging the implicit bias that women are less worthy of the same educational opportunities provided to men. It is undeniable that socioeconomics, geographical locations, family belief system, and many other factors contribute to considerable disparities in education. However, patriarchal systems rationalize this denial of opportunity and support the notion that men are more capable of exerting power, and women's subordinate positions in all areas of society are justified. This obsolete yet consistent perspective impacts educational equality and creates discrepancies for women on national and international levels.

Lack of clarity on women's issues – We must recognize that all issues related to the financial systems, environmental issues, fundamental reforms to the criminal justice system, and even national security are all women's issues. However, in the US, women are not an integral part of the decision-making group to tackle these critical challenges. It is essential to recognize that women in power bring a different perspective for grassroots changes in any society. Out of 193 countries, the United States ranks 75th regarding women's representation in government (Women in National Parliaments, 2019). Even though not including women in the political system is a global issue, the US, despite making some strides since 2018, still has a long way to go.

Economic disparities, sexism, and racism – The compelling mixture of sexism, racism, and economic inequality impacts women both in the US and globally and is the consequence of the massive systemic power imbalances. In the United States, economic inequality is unique in the sense that it is both racialized and gendered, with Black and Latina women constantly making less than any other groups, and therefore, staying at the far end of the economic order. Moreover, compared to White men and women and other racial groups, Black and Latina women often have less desirable jobs, with lower incomes and higher poverty rates. The federal government has a central role in structuring such inequality, specifically, with public policies promoting racial inequities impacting women more than other groups. These policies often have unfair consequences for marginalized women since federal-level assessments about investing resources have vastly different effects centered around women's race and ethnicity. Thus, in analyzing the economic status of minority women, we need to use an intersectional lens for the economic inequality linking public policies and economic outcomes.

Trauma-centered feminism – Women in the US may have enjoyed more freedom and better health than many women in other countries. Still, young women are vulnerable, fragile, and in imminent danger on many college campuses. Thus, a new trauma-centered feminist movement does not focus on equality with men. It is focusing on protecting women from men. Wulfhorst (2018), as part of the Thompson Reuters Foundation, published a study revealing that the US was one of the top ten most dangerous countries in the world for women. There were attempts to show that this study was not scientific, and the survey looked at experts' perceptions and not actual data, which is very problematic. Nevertheless, the US continues to promote the idea that it is a haven for women. The media promotes that women in the US enjoy more freedom than women in other countries, which is part of the hegemonic colonial way of looking at the world, which never helps with making progress on issues related to women and their everyday experiences.

Access to equal opportunity – Globally, many women would like their daughters to be more educated even in the middle of a war, conflict, or crisis because it would provide their daughters with opportunities they were denied. Nevertheless, even when women have access to educational opportunities in the US and globally, many women still lack equal access to economic and educational opportunities. More women go to college than men, but it is harder for them to pay back student loans because of the unequal pay. More women are working at minimum-wage jobs than men, and the minimum wage cannot keep a mother and her child above the poverty line. Many mothers cannot even afford to work to build their future because they cannot find low-cost childcare options for their children. Thus, regardless of women's progress in the US, opportunities are still fundamentally defined by gender.

The US has recently elected a large number of women as congressional representatives. If we want women to achieve more equality, we need women leaders and advocates to acknowledge the danger of inaction. We need women and men in South Sudan and the South Side of Chicago to demand quality education for their daughters. Women leaders and advocates, and congressional leaders, who have advanced due to the collective effort of so many, should challenge the system and keep the doors of opportunity open for other women. They need to make sure every girl and every woman has the chance to lead life to her fullest potential.

Not honoring caregiving – Women in the United States and globally provide care for children, parents, spouses, siblings, and extended family members while often holding on to more than one full-time job and competing with men who have only one job. In the US, over half of the women are the primary breadwinners in their households. The typical discussion has been around how women should persuade men to "help" more. However, we need a paradigm shift and to think differently about valuing caregiving. We must perceive providing care as work. Women provide physical care, teach new skills, provide coaching, mentoring, and advising, which is very time-consuming and essential but can be as rewarding as many other types of jobs that have pay attached to them. We need to put a higher economic value on caregiving by compensating women far more by government and private funding. We also need to honor their contributions socially by enhancing the stature and respect for caregiving and care careers. Fundamentally, we need to perceive traditional women's work as genuinely identical to classic men's work.

Traversing professional life and motherhood – Balancing work and family life is a significant challenge facing working women in the US. Working mothers can either lean on their careers to have a sense of identity or rely on motherhood to have emotional fulfillment but can rarely rely on both. Women should be able to return to work after being away due to parenting demands, but adequate maternity leave is still a major issue. Even developing countries have been able to navigate and deal with issues related to maternity leave successfully compared to the US. The Organization for Economic Co-operation and Development (OECD) or the European Union (EU) Family Database have focused on two key policies: childcare leave for parents and early childhood education and care for preschool children. They reviewed these policies in the 41 high- and middle-income countries. The US was the only nation offering absolutely no national paid leave with zero weeks.

Rise of maternal mortality – One of the biggest challenges women in the US and worldwide face today is increasing maternal mortality rates. According to the World Health Organization (2019), 830 women die every day from pregnancy-related causes that could have been avoidable. These numbers are way higher in developing countries and among women of color in the United States. Black women in the US are particularly the most affected, at a ratio of 25.1 deaths per 100,000 (Vilda *et al.*, 2019). Furthermore, between 1980 and 1990, this ratio did not improve for black women, and they have not improved since then. These disparities happen because the US is a racially divided society. Black women are suffering from higher levels of stress and marginalization, causing higher rates of health issues that are often unrecognized and can potentially lead to preventable deaths.

Misogyny normalized – For the past few years, women in America have suffered the consequences of normalized misogyny, which puts women's rights in real jeopardy. It began with a president with a serious record of making appalling and humiliating assertions about women. Conceivably, even worse, his administration has converted these misogynous stances into specific actions. For instance, despite the growth of the MeToo movement, the Department of Education has introduced measures to provide greater protections by weakening Title IX (Napolitano, 2018). The 44th US president also suspended a federal rule to close the gender and race gap pay, which is harmful to minorities and working women and their families.

In summary, better education, greater health and safety, and more political representation will empower women and girls to contribute to the health and productivity of their families, communities, and countries, creating a ripple effect that benefits everyone. Thus, the best solution for expanding peace, equality, and security moving forward, is to give intelligent, vigorous, and strong women a seat at the decision-making table, both at home and around the world.

The Healing Power of Psychotherapy

As discussed in this chapter, gender and gender differences are not innately problematic. However, we experience many problems when gender becomes the marker for well-regarded and devalued. In almost all cultures worldwide, males and masculine attributes are preferred, valued, and associated with power (Brown, 2010). This section will introduce empowerment feminist therapy (EFT) as one of the most suitable psychotherapeutic modalities to help women. The critical value of this model is in integrating multicultural and social justice perspectives with female-centered therapy (Remer & Oh, 2013). Earlier models were not inclusive and centered mainly on helping White middle-class and upper-class women. This EFT model focuses on examining biases and integrating multicultural viewpoints, which increases its pertinence and usefulness with men and women from many different walks of life (Díaz-Lázaro *et al.*, 2012). In this model, all forms of oppression are identified, and women's diverse personal and social identities are recognized (Worell & Remer, 2003). The primary objective is to transform toxic and harmful social systems and support individuals to control the relational and systemic issues affecting their welfare (Worell & Remer, 2003). In this model, clients' past, current, and future suffering and distress and their power and resiliency with coping are emphasized (Herlihy & Corey, 2013; Remer & Oh, 2013). The EFT model should be used with men and women of all genders and ages, and both male and female psychotherapists must utilize it. This approach also helps men and boys articulate their emotions freely and accept their own sense of self as well as have a better relationship with women and girls. Specifically, it is crucial for male psychotherapists to adopt feminist therapy and impact their clients and society in fundamentally meaningful ways. This means that they have to be conscious about their own privilege and use their power to challenge sexism and other types of oppression (Herlihy & Corey, 2013). Empowering feminist therapy can be very useful and practical with adolescents in order to provide an empowering substitute for understanding their developmental challenges (Lovell, 2016). The EFT model has been used with many different groups, including older adults and caregivers, to fight against depression and increase the quality of life (Stripling, 2016); men who have abused women (Herlihy & Corey, 2013); women of color facing poverty, trauma, and oppression (East & Roll, 2015); immigrant women (Díaz-Lázaro et al., 2012); treatment of eating disorders (Pollack, 2003); sex education curriculum (Askew, 2007); healing for survivors of intimate partner violence (Crowder, 2016); tackling relational aggression (Brown, 2013); and conceptualizing adolescence development (Otting & Prosek, 2016).

Empowering Feminist Therapy Principles

Empowering feminist therapy's focus is on gender, social location, and power with the aim of liberation and social change (Herlihy & Corey, 2013). As part of the therapeutic process, the influence and power of socialization in the clients' lives are examined (Díaz-Lázaro et al., 2012). This model attempts to evaluate the strong relationships between the internal and external, individual and society, and experiences and environmental contexts to show the influence of culture and environment at the global, institutional, relational, biological, and spiritual levels. According to Brown (2010), the fundamental tenets of empowerment feminist therapy are based on critical consciousness and devotion to social change, an equal relationship between the therapist and the client, and a strength-based approach to reexamine psychological suffering. The original feminist ideology that "personal is political" is at the center of this approach because it examines the reciprocal impact of our lives, our belief systems, and our social values, honoring the intersectionality of our diverse selves (Remer & Oh, 2013). The EFT therapist is conscious of the power differential in the therapy room and treats the client as the expert, focusing on the client's sense of self and the level of awareness to make fundamental change possible.

EFT Therapy Techniques

The empowering therapy model is an action-oriented theory attempting to transform philosophy into practice (Evans et al., 2011). It requires the therapist to be self-reflective and conscious about their preconceived notions creating a safe context for the clients to reevaluate their experiences (Crowder, 2016; Evans et al., 2011). The following section describes some techniques utilized by the EFT therapists:

Cultural analysis – It involves helping clients to recognize all the specific messages they have internalized about gender roles evaluating the effects of these internalized beliefs on their emotional, cognitive, and behavioral reactions. The next phase is making a conscious decision to hold on to some of these messages and get rid of others. The last phase is to create a concrete plan to carry out some of these changes (Remer & Oh, 2013). The therapist can use reflective questions, such as: "What messages did you receive when you were growing up, and how do they impact you now?"; "Where did those messages come from (e.g., parents, teachers, media)?"; "What gendered expectations are you measuring yourself against and possibly trying to live up to?"; "What are the potential negative or positive effects of this?"; "Which messages do you want to keep, and which do you want to change?"; and "How will you do it?" (Evans *et al.*, 2011; Remer & Oh, 2013). The goal is to help clients become aware of these internalized messages and intentionally decide to disregard the harmful ones and their relationships. Further, the presenting issues and client's life experiences are viewed based on power dynamics in the relationship because the unbalanced access to power in society influences women's lives (Ballou *et al.*, 2008).

Power analysis – Another technique utilized by EFT therapists is assessing the inequality of power in society amongst men and women and how it affects access to resources and impacts women's self-confidence (Herlihy & Corey, 2013). It is highly critical to include discourses about the impact of sexism, racism, and other forms of discrimination as part of the therapeutic process (Remer & Oh, 2013). Similar to the gender analysis, clients must assess their contexts and see the impact of relational power on their relationships and all parts of their lives, including work and family dynamics. It is critical to validate the client's lived experiences so they can feel supported in their attempt to gain more access to power. This intervention provides clients with a sense of social awareness, so they can purposefully and consciously decide to take in or refuse prevalent and harmful societal messages.

Gender-role intervention – This technique includes framing personal concerns within the context of collective messages and expectations in any given society by using reframing to help women shift their focus from emotional and inter-nalized experiences to societal messages (Díaz-Lázaro *et al.*, 2012). This is helpful because it considers external factors contributing to a problem, which helps with the client's therapeutic growth and self-esteem (Herlihy & Corey, 2013). It is also beneficial because it allows the therapist to challenge clients' self-defeating behaviors, linking them to more extensive societal issues instead of individual failings and inadequacies (Evans *et al.*, 2011). Symptoms are reframed as proper tactics for coping and normal responses to the environ-mental context (Evans *et al.*, 2011). For example, adolescent girls are often labeled as shallow and too focused on appearances. However, we don't often talk about how women are flooded with strong messages about the importance of their looks and how these messages become way more explicit when they become adolescents.

Relabeling – The EFT therapists utilize the original family therapy technique of relabeling to focus on the positive aspects of clients' character or behavior instead of focusing on the negatives (Remer & Oh, 2013). For example, clients' "sensitivity" is relabeled as being mindful and conscious about the feelings of others and their own, which is a precious attribute in relationships and in expressing self and relating to others.

Strength-based assessment and exercise – Women often have some challenging life experiences that they feel powerless about, but unconsciously, they handle them with resilience and strength. However, society does not train women to assess these experiences as positive and life-changing. One helpful exercise is asking clients to reflect on a difficult life circumstance from their past but concentrate on the strength that helped them overcome it and thrive in that situation instead of getting stuck in processing the pain and suffering. As they verbally identify their strengths, the therapist can highlight and reconceptualize their experience as a foundation for other aspects of their lives. These strength-based exercises help women recognize their resilience, power, and strength.

Assertiveness training – This type of training provides women with specific psychoeducational information about the distinct differences between being assertive, aggressive, or exhibiting passive behaviors. The EFT therapist can use role-plays to help women practice proper conflict resolution techniques to gain confidence and manage their own relational issues.

Advocacy – The most salient hallmark of feminist therapy is to use and model for clients how to advocate for themselves and others. "The personal is political" is the main principle of the feminist perspective, which is based on the idea that personal change only happens when we directly contribute to the political and social action or change (Evans *et al.*, 2011). Based on the empowerment feminist therapy principles, clients are encouraged and empowered to become change agents and exercise their assertiveness and advocacy skills in meaningful ways that make sense to them. The therapy room must be a safe space to assess and critique gendered-based messages and feel confident to advocate for self and others in developing critical consciousness (Clonan-Roy, Jacobs, & Nakkula, 2016).

Group work – The EFT model has been successful and influential in group settings because it connects women with each other to share resources and help each other with emotional growth (Herlihy & Corey, 2013).

Bibliotherapy – This is always helpful and can be utilized in any therapeutic setting so clients can use it to educate themselves as well as others in their lives. The therapist can suggest books, blogs, documentaries, and websites to find more information and gain more knowledge about specific topics. Research reveals that bibliotherapy can have a powerful therapeutic impact and help clients' satisfaction (Herlihy & Corey, 2013).

Summary

Psychotherapists should integrate the EFT model into their practice to focus on consciousness, liberation, identity exploration, and internalized social and cultural messages that cause pain and suffering. The empowerment feminist therapy does not pathologize relational difficulties and frames them as coping strategies or survival techniques (Herlihy & Corey, 2013). Like many other family therapy models, feminist psychotherapists do not use diagnosis. They believe that it dehumanizes the client and blames the individual behavior instead of the social system that creates these difficulties. If a diagnosis is necessary, the psychotherapist must explain that the diagnosis does not become internalized and support stereotypes. It is always critical to evaluate and assess clients' environment and not get stuck with their symptoms. For example, personality disorders instead of PTSD have long been used to diagnose women with a history of trauma and abuse. While the therapy process is fundamentally hierarchical, as was mentioned before, a collaborative and power-neutral relationship in the therapy room can be beneficial. The psychotherapists have to be in a grounded place with their own self of the therapist explorations and take a very non-defensive and open stance in order to reduce the power differential, act as nonexpert, and build trust. The entire therapy process should be collaborative from the first diagnostic session to treatment planning and termination. The self of the therapist training should help the psychotherapist to use self-disclosure to discuss experiences with gender and oppression in order to normalize women's experiences with gender-related issues. The psychotherapist must be very careful to use self-disclosure only to benefit the client and not get distracted from the process. Further, feminist psychotherapists must be incessantly self-reflective and conscious about not imposing their own values. They must create a safe environment so clients can process their feelings, search for appropriate options, and be motivated to choose for themselves. Although women share many personal and relational challenges due to the gender dynamics in any society, it is imperative to discuss specific issues impacting women with different sexual orientations. The following section will discuss some of the challenges lesbians face and how psychotherapy can help them overcome them.

Special Considerations in Working with Lesbian Relationships

Many aspects of same-sex and heterosexual couples' relationships are the same. However, due to the vast differences in their social context and the strong influences of the dominant heterosexual culture as well as traditional expectations of gender dynamics in their relationships, they may experience a tremendous level of distress. They may have to deal with a lack of support in many aspects of their lives, including family, legal, religious, economic systems, and lack of social support. Societal prejudices add to their stress level, and since women have learned to internalize their pain, the lesbian couple may suffer the consequences of this internalization even more. Given the level of negative contextual factors, it is impressive that lesbian couples have stable relationships and show a high level of resiliency. The following sections delve into the unique challenges for lesbian couples, so psychotherapists can better understand these issues and help these couples' relationships flourish.

Relationship expectation – The quality of time couples spend together, and the level of emotional support they expect from each other can be a source of tension in any relationship. However, for lesbian couples who have been socialized as women to be responsible for relational, emotional support, it can create even more tension. Psychotherapists should first tackle women's socialization issues before discussing relationship expectations for lesbian couples.

Habitual behaviors – Women in heterosexual couples' relationships often complain about their pet peeves and the annoying habits of their male partners. However, when these habits are repeated in lesbian relationships, it becomes a source of tension because now, both members of the couple are annoyed with each other over these minor issues. Some examples are leaving drawers open on a dresser, displaying road rage, leaving the light on in different parts of the house; speaking loudly; being late for events; forgetting significant milestones in the relationship; losing important documents, not checking mail, or not answering emails on time. It is helpful to normalize the reactions to these annoyances and then reframe them as human behavior instead of gendered specific behaviors.

Sex and intimacy – Having conflicts over sexual intimacy is part of many couple relational dynamics. Couples' therapy routinely discusses issues related to frequency and mismatched sexual desires. However, since lesbian couples have been socialized not to initiate sexual intimacy, these issues can create unavoidable tension. Psychotherapy can help lesbian couples become aware of these gendered patterns and consciously change their socialization. The other socialization-based dynamic is agreeing to have sex just to please the partner, which over time creates more conflict. Lesbian couples should be helped make a conscious effort to develop healthy intimacy and then be sexual.

Household chores – It makes sense that couples start fighting about living together as soon as they start living together because being under one roof always requires new rules, guidelines, flexibility, and compromise. For lesbian couples, this becomes more complicated because women have been socialized to take care of household chores more than the male partner. Still, they want to renegotiate their division of tasks. Psychotherapists must help lesbian couples use fairness and relational justice to balance the demands of household chores.

Friendships and jealousy – Sometimes, couples' relationships will enhance or deteriorate based on their friendships with others. Couples may deal with trust issues and jealousy, and they may think that their partner is cheating. Lesbian couples may need to deal with these issues even more because their union was not recognized by law until recently, making it easier to change relationship status without significant financial and emotional consequences. Additionally, bisexual women may have to deal with more tension in their relationships because the partner may worry about competing with both men and women. This may be a greater source of conflict in newer relationships than older ones as well as in non-monogamous and open relationships. Psychotherapy can successfully help these couples by validating their perspectives and normalizing social patterns and helping them negotiate relationship boundaries based on fairness and equality for both.

Financial issues – One of the main conflicts in committed relationships is managing finances. This may include stress and tension about one person making more money. One partner may be unemployed, have disagreements about spending, savings, or tight finances. These concerns are more stressful for lesbian couples because women earn less than men and are more likely to support themselves due to cut-off relationships from family. Educational information about how financial issues impact all couples' relationships can be used as a foundation to discuss lesbian couples' issues and encourage them to problem-solve together and remember to be flexible and compromise.

Dealing with relatives – Arguing over relationships with relatives is another typical relational issue for all couples. Many couples have conflicts over invisible loyalties to the family of origin, how to handle a toxic family member and many forms of cultural conflicts. However, in lesbian relationships, lack of familiar support and perhaps homophobic reactions can become a natural source of tension. Psychotherapy sessions can be organized around some family of origin work and socialization that can influence people's reactions to lesbian couples. Working on differentiation and trying not to take things too personally, and having the flexibility to renegotiate relationship boundaries can be very helpful to strengthen lesbian couples' bonds and enhance their coping skills.

Health – Lesbians more than straight women have mental and physical health issues (Autostraddle Grown-Ups survey, 2015). This can be related to many factors, including feeling isolated due to their relationship being viewed as nonnormative, trying to fit in, and being stressed out about not being accepted by family and friends. It is apparent that lack of emotional health contributes to physical fitness, and then they both contribute to a lack of well-being. Psychotherapy should help lesbian couples become conscious of the impact of stressors and try to reduce their emotional stress by exercising, healthy eating, and mindfulness, which will positively impact their physical health. Teaching lesbian couples healthy coping skills can also contribute to their overall health.

Political and social justice issues – The feminist mantra that "the personal is political" can become a source of tension for lesbian couples. For example, their relations would be highly affected when one partner is White and does not fully understand the issues that may impact the nonwhite partner. In some situations, experiences of racism and discrimination can greatly trouble one partner without processing and complaining about it within the context of the relationship. Psychotherapy can be helpful for lesbian couples to understand that political and social justice issues are often deeply tied to personality and not part of the relationship dynamics. This means that couples can evaluate these belief systems and act based on their own values. Further, since the political and social issues are not directly linked to the relational conflicts, it becomes less of a problem in long-term relationships. Over time, couples learn to compromise and perhaps even change their views on political views.

Parenting and raising children – Girls are socialized to grow up and become mothers from an early age. The expectations that they need to be good mothers are continuously part of their conscious and unconscious thinking. One of the sources of tension for heterosexual couples is related to raising children and how they need to work together and not against each other to raise emotionally and physically healthy children. Men are often blamed for making mistakes in child-rearing, and they often feel defensive when they seek couples therapy about issues related to their children. The same dynamics exist for lesbian couples, except that both partners think they may know everything about raising children due to their early socialization. They may unconsciously try to one-up the other partner. When lesbian couples seek therapy to resolve issues related to parenting, it is imperative to discuss their socialization patterns. Therapists can teach them how to use these skills collaboratively instead of having a competition about who is more nurturing and emotionally available for children.

Conclusion

Across the world, there is still this persistent question about whether girls and women as a group continue to experience oppression. It is undeniable that there have been positive changes for women globally. However, there is still enormous inequality for women in the United States and worldwide. For example, globally, violence against women and girls, unequal pay, lack of access to education, and the unbalanced number of men in positions of power are impacting women and girls' everyday experiences (Crawford & Unger, 2004). Evans *et al.* (2011) explain that the "oppression of women/girls transcends culture" (p. 91). They discuss some examples of female oppression in the United States, such as the high numbers of women and girls facing sexual assault and harassment; lower salaries in primarily female fields like teaching and nursing; a much lower number of females in positions of power; more domestic obligations at home regardless of employment status; and unfairness in education and mental health toward women.

Notwithstanding many societal advancements, sexism is still very prevalent in almost every aspect of our lives. The mere fact that someone is a female makes them more susceptible to violence, poverty, and rights violations. Overall, a report reviewing family-friendly policies in 41 countries by the OECD used country-level indicators such as duration of paid leave for mothers and fathers and low-cost daycare centers for children. The result of the study revealed that Iceland, Norway, and Sweden hold the top three places in offering family-friendly policies. Many other countries struggle to have consistent family-friendly policies. Here are some suggestions to improve women and girls' lives cross-culturally with public policies that can be discussed and promoted in the therapy rooms:

- Provide fundamental education about the impact of sexual abuse and pass enforceable laws that protect women and children against any kinds of sexual abuse and human trafficking.

- Provide impactful education about the damaging aspects of violence in long-term relationships and pass enforceable laws against intimate partner violence.
- Educate both men and women about their significant responsibilities toward an unborn child and hold men accountable for their contribution in making a baby instead of having only women responsible for parenting responsibilities and abortion.
- Provide legal and nationwide paid leave to both mothers and fathers so they can equally feel responsible for raising their children.
- Provide resources for mothers and fathers to also be able to have child-care leave.
- Provide all children access to high-quality, inexpensive, and available child-care centers regardless of family income.
- Ensure that mothers can breastfeed by providing such things as a room to pump and store milk, guaranteed breastfeeding breaks, and quality child-care close to work.
- Collect continuous data on all aspects of family-friendly policies to make sure these policies are monitored, compared and all countries held accountable.

References

Askew, J. (2007). Breaking the taboo: An exploration of female university students' experiences of attending a feminist-informed sex education course. *Sex Education: Sexuality, Society and Learning, 7*(3), 251–264. doi:10.1080/14681810701448051

Autostraddle Grown-Ups survey. (2015, October 8). *Gal Pals, Community, Money, Marriage, Bike-riding and Acceptance Make LGBTQ Women Feel Healthier.* Autostraddle. https://www.autostraddle.com/gal-pals-community-money-marriage-bike-riding-and-acceptance-make-lgbtq-women-feel-healthier-295603/

Ballou, M., Hill, M., & West, C. (2008). *Feminist Therapy Theory and Practice: A Contemporary Perspective.* New York: Springer.

Brown, L. S. (2010). *Feminist Therapy.* Washington, DC: American Psychological Association.

Brown, L. S. (2013). Feminist therapy as a path to friendship with women. *Women and Therapy, 36*(1–2), 11–22. doi:10.1080/02703149.2012.720556

Clonan-Roy, K., Jacobs, C. E., & Nakkula, M. J. (2016). Towards a model of positive youth development specific to girls of color: Perspectives on development, resilience, and empowerment. *Gender Issues, 33*(2), 96–121. doi:10.1007/s12147-016-9156-7

Crawford, M., & Unger, R. (2004). *Women and Gender: A Feminist Psychology.* (4th ed.). Boston, MA: McGraw-Hill.

Crowder, R. (2016). Mindfulness based feminist therapy: The intermingling edges of self compassion and social justice. *Journal of Religion and Spirituality in Social Work: Social Thought, 35*(1–2), 24–40. doi:10.1080/15426432.2015.1080605

Díaz-Lázaro, C. M., Verdinelli, S., & Cohen, B. B. (2012). Empowerment feminist therapy with Latina immigrants: Honoring the complexity and socio-cultural contexts of clients' lives. *Women and Therapy, 35*(1–2), 80–92. doi:10.1080/02703149.2012.634730

East, J. F., & Roll, S. J. (2015). Women, poverty, and trauma: An Empowerment Practice approach. *Social Work, 60*(4), 279–286. http://www.jstor.org/stable/24881177

Evans, K. M., Kincade, E. A., & Seem, S. R. (2011). *Introduction to Feminist Therapy: Strategies for Social and Individual Change.* Los Angeles, CA: Sage.

Hausmann, R., Tyson, L. D., & Zahidi, S. (2010). *The Global Gender Gap Report.* Geneva: World Economic Forum.

Herlihy, B., & Corey, G. (2013). Feminist therapy. In G. Corey (Ed.), *Theory and Practice of Counseling and Psychotherapy* (9th ed., pp. 360–394). Belmont, CA: Brooks/Cole, Cengage Learning.

Lovell, K. (2016). Girls are equal too: Education, body politics, and the making of teenage feminism. *Gender Issues, 33*(2), 71–95. doi:10.1007/s12147-016-9155-8

Napolitano, J. (2018). Don't let the Trump administration undermine Title IX. *The Washington Post.* Retrieved online at https://www.washingtonpost.com.

OECD (2018). *Investing in Women and Girls.* https://www.oecd.org/dac/gender-deve lopment/45704694.pdf

Otting, T. L., & Prosek, E. A. (2016). Integrating feminist therapy and expressive arts with adolescent clients. *Journal of Creativity in Mental Health, 11*(1), 78–89. doi:10.1080/ 15401383.2015.1019167

Pollack, D. (2003). Pro-eating disorder websites: What should be the feminist response? *Feminism and Psychology, 13*(2), 246–251. doi:10.1177/0959353503013002008

Remer, P. A., & Oh, K. H. (2013). Feminist therapy in counseling psychology. In C. Z. Enns & E. N. Williams (Eds), *The Oxford Handbook of FReminist Multicultural Counseling Psychology* (pp. 304–321). New York, NY: Oxford University Press.

Sedgh, G., Ashford, L. S., & Hussain, R. (2016). *Unmet Need for Contraception in Developing Countries: Examining Women's Reasons for Not Using a Method.* New York: Guttmacher Institute, https://www.guttmacher.org/report/unmet-need-for-contraception-in-dev eloping-countries

Singh, G. K. (2010). *Maternal Mortality in the United States, 1935–2007: Substantial Racial/ Ethnic, Socioeconomic, and Geographic Disparities Persist.* A 75th Anniversary Publication. Health Resources and Services Administration, Maternal and Child Health Bureau. https://www.hrsa.gov/sites/default/files/ourstories/mchb75th/mchb75matern almortality.pdf

Singh, G. K., & Stella, M. Y. (2019). Infant mortality in the United States, 1915–1917: Large social inequalities have persisted for over a century. *International Journal of Maternal and Child Health and AIDS, 8*(1), 19. https://www.ncbi.nlm.nih.gov/ pmc/articles/PMC6487507/

Stripling, A. M. (2016). The healthy aging group: A proposed treatment model for societal & individual aging empowerment. *Women and Therapy, 39*(1–2), 124–140. doi:10.1080/02703149.2016.1116324

UNICEF &WSSCC. (2005). Women, Water and Hygiene, Are Key to Change in Africa. *Press release, 14.* http://www.unicef.org/media/media_28260.html.

United Nation (2020). Make this the century of women's equality: UN chief. https:// news.un.org/en/story/2020/02/1058271

UN Women. (2020). *Facts and Figures: Women's Leadership and Political Participation..* https:// www.unwomen.org/en/what-we-do/leadership-and-political-participation/facts-and-figures#notes

Vilda, D., Wallace, M., Dyer, L., Harville, E., & Theall, K. (2019). Income inequality and racial disparities in pregnancy-related mortality in the US. *SSM - Population Health, 9*, 100477 https://doi: 10.1016/j.ssmph.2019.100477

Wills., A., Smith. J., and Hicks, C. (2019). *All the countries that had a woman leader before the U.S.* CNN. https://www.cnn.com/interactive/2016/06/politics/women-world-leaders/

Women in National Parliaments: World classifcation. (2019). http://archive.ipu.org/wmn-e/classif.htm

Worell, J., & Remer, P. (2003). *Feminist Perspectives in Therapy: Empowering Diverse Women* (2nd ed.). Hoboken, NJ: John Wiley.

World Health Organization (2013). *Violence Against Women: A 'global health problem of epidemic proportions.' New Clinical and Policy Guidelines Launched to Guide Health Sector Response.* https://www.who.int/mediacentre/news/releases/2013/violence_against_women_20130620/en

World Health Organization (2016, October 13). *Strategies Towards Ending Preventable Maternal Mortality (EPMM).* Geneva: World Health Organization. https://www.who.int/reproductivehealth/topics/maternal_perinatal/epmm/en/

World Health Organization. (2019). *Maternal Mortality.* https://www.who.int/newsroom/fact-sheets/detail/maternal-mortality

World Health Organization (2020). *Child Marriages: 39000 every day.* https://www.who.int/mediacentre/news/releases/2013/child_marriage_20130307/en/

World Health Organization. (2020). *Female Genital Mutliation.* World Health Organization. https://www.who.int/en/news-room/fact-sheets/detail/female-genital-mutilation.

Wulfhorst, E. (2018). *Exclusive: US among 10 Most Dangerous Countries for Women amid #MeToo Campaign – Poll.* Reuters. https://www.reuters.com/article/us-women-dangerous-poll-usa-exclusive/exclusive-u-s-among-10-most-dangerous-countries-for-women-amid-metoo-campaign-poll-idUSKBN1JM02G

4 The Impact of Colonization on Global Social Justice

Introduction

According to the Merriam-Webster Dictionary, colonialism is defined as "controlled by one power over a dependent area or people." More specifically, colonialism is about one or more nations or countries overpowering and suppressing other countries: dominating its population, using its natural and human resources while imposing its own language and cultural values on the people of the country they conquered. By 1914, a large majority of the world's nations were colonized by European governments (Ferrante, 2007). The concepts of colonialism and imperialism are closely linked to the policy or tenet of utilizing force and power to control another nation or people perfectly under imperialism and colonialism. However, the word colony comes from the Latin word *colonia*, which means farm or state. This indicates that the practice of colonialism usually included transferring people from their own homes to a new territory. At the same time, the colonizers and settlers lived permanently on the indigenous people's lands and maintained political and cultural commitment and loyalty to their country of origin. Imperialism, however, comes from the Latin term *imperium*, which means order and control. Therefore, the term imperialism defines one country as overpowering another, whether through settlement, dominance, or any ancillary mechanisms of control (Kohn & Reddy, 2017).

Colonialism History

Big empires like Ancient Greece, Ancient Rome, Ancient Egypt, and Phoenicia practiced colonialism in ancient times. These civilizations stretched their borders to utilize the resources of other nations starting around 1550 BC. They formed colonies to capture the physical and human resources of the people they overpowered to spread their control. Modern colonialism began during the Age of Discovery in the fifteenth century when Portugal started looking for new trade routes outside of Europe. The Portuguese colonial empire was the first and the last European empire that started from the conquest of Ceuta in 1415, and then Morocco, North Africa, and continued until the formal

DOI: 10.4324/9781003088189-5

surrender of Macau to the People's Republic of China in 1999 (Bandeira Jerónimo, 2018). Soon after, Portugal's competing nation, Spain, searched for new lands. In 1492, Christopher Columbus started exploring a western route to India and China (Bandeira Jerónimo, 2018). However, he landed in the Bahamas, which was the beginning of the power of the Spanish and Portuguese empires in the Americas, India, Africa, and Asia. In the meantime, England, the Netherlands, France, and Germany started building their own empires abroad, battling Spain and Portugal over the lands they had already dominated and occupied. In the eighteenth and nineteenth centuries, many of these colonies managed to earn independence starting with the American Revolution in 1776, and the Haitian Revolution in 1781. Nonetheless, the eastern half of the world continued to attract European colonial powers. They started taking over African lands, fighting each other to access these nations' natural resources, and establishing colonies until the decolonization beginning around 1914 to 1975 (Bandeira Jerónimo, 2018).

From the late nineteenth century until the end of World War II, all powerful nations globally followed imperialist strategies to reach national, political, and economic gains. History reveals that just between 1885 and 1914, European countries added 2.8 billion hectares to their colonial territories (*Columbia Electronic Encyclopedia*, 2013). Later on, the United States and Japan decided to join the European countries to create their own empires. Therefore, almost all of Africa was under colonial control and dominance, and the British Empire alone dominated one-quarter of the world's population. It is critical to note that occupied lands utilized by colonial countries significantly differed across time and space in different locations. Some became colonies that the new incomers settled, and colonizers established considerably vast and long-lasting communities. Some territories had raw resources that needed to be extricated or were strategically located and controlled by military forces using indigenous people controlled by colonial officials. These colonial societies intensely impacted occupiers and the occupied lands' economic, social, cultural, and political systems.

Rationale for Colonizing and the Power of Resistance

European colonial powers defended and justified their invasions of indigenous peoples' lands by declaring that taking over these nations was based on their legal and religious duties. They claimed that occupying the land and destroying the culture of indigenous peoples were justified because the colonizers' role was to civilize "barbaric" or "savage" nations, and they had the best interests of those whose lands and peoples they exploited in mind (Kohn & Reddy, 2017). It is critical to note that indigenous people continuously tried to resist the efforts of the colonizers who occupied the lands they already owned and populated. Thus, defiance and opposition through violent and nonviolent means have been fundamental parts of the story of colonialism in different continents.

Costs and Benefits of Colonization

Colonial governments claimed they provided foundations for better roads and accommodations and distributed medical and technological awareness and information. In some situations, they even supported literacy among indigenous people. They also claimed that through the adoption of Western human rights ideas, they created democratic governmental systems (Mani, 1987). Nevertheless, intimidation, cruelty, racism, political repression, economic exploitation, and involuntary assimilation were directly linked to any benefits. Colonialism's impacts also include environmental deprivation, the spread of disease, financial instability, ethnic conflicts, and human rights violations (Blanton *et al.*, 2001; Conklin, 1998) lasting way longer than the colonial occupations in these counties.

Relation between Gender and Colonialism

Researchers have long realized that these global colonial systems were sustained and justified, at least partly, using language and policies grounded on gender ideals. This set of gender ideals integrated principles about the proper sexual behaviors of men and women and marked differences between colonizing and indigenous cultures. The same applied to racial differences to show the inherent inequality of colonized and indigenous people. These gender-based politics were not the same in all colonies. They differed based on prevailing indigenous cultures, the existence of natural resources, the presence of colonial settlers, the impact on the global economy, and access to lands. Specific beliefs about gender, sexuality, and gender roles somehow legitimized and preserved differences between colonizers and the colonized since it helped colonizers classify and consequently divide indigenous peoples.

It seems very apparent that the colonizing system rationalized the imbalanced allocation of power between colonizers and colonized and justified the presence of colonies. The main source of justification was related to colonized men's and women's sexual behaviors, desires, and manners. For example, in French Indochina, British India, the Dutch East Indies, and British South Africa, colonizers planted the idea that White women were in persistent threat from colonized men's insatiable and tenacious sexual cravings. Thus, they justified strict separation between the indigenous people and the colonizers and controlled both White women and colonized people to protect White women from supposedly being raped. Consequently, White women living in colonies were ironically comfortable but controlled and restricted by White men.

Furthermore, colonized men could not ever be in a position to have any decision-making power over White women and were routinely excluded from these positions and had to endure severe punishment if they ever crossed the boundaries between themselves and colonizing women. For example, in India, a decision was made to permit Indian judges' jurisdiction over some European cases. However, British colonizers strongly resisted this suggestion. They stated that Indians could not assert judgment over Europeans and seriously attacked the bill because they claimed that it endangered the safety of White women even though the bill had nothing to do with women. They asserted that Indian men had the fantasy of possessing White women, and since they treated their own women so poorly, they could not be trusted to be judges. This opposition helped drop the bill, and Indian men were kept strictly subordinate, using gender to overpower the colonized men.

Interestingly enough, since there were few White women in many of these colonies, which helped keep White men in the colonized areas, the colonizers encouraged sexual relationships with colonized women. These indigenous women had fewer expenses than European women and were expected to take care of domestic duties as well as provide sexual satisfaction without the legal protections or any kinds of marital rights. Soon, mixed-race children that were the results of these relationships could not be classified in any category. By the 1880s, concubinage was the most common domestic arrangement for European men. This created tens of thousands of mixed-race children, creating a blur in dividing the colonizers and the colonized. In these instances, the colonizers' officials increasingly began to argue that these women did not have the skills or the morals to raise these mixed-race children who were not worthy of European citizenship. Later on, the colonizers encouraged White women to immigrate to these colonies to marry White settlers. At the same time, prostitution became another means for sexual satisfaction for White men who could not afford to bring White women to the colony. Thus, the gendered patterns of sexual and family relationships continued to be one of the central tenets of the colonizers' relationship with the colonized.

Furthermore, the colonizers divided the colonized based on how they liked their docile and compliant behavior and how they treated women. Over time, they created a drift and separation between the colonized themselves. These perceptions of group and gendered differences highly reinvigorated the privileged and superior treatment of one group. It also imposed a rigorous division between two indigenous groups and deeply impacted the colonizers' relationship with the colonized. In fact, the way colonizers used language to describe gender differences in colonizing situations served to maintain distinctions between colonizer and colonized and strictly preserved colonizer-centered disparities between different groups of colonized people.

Gender and the Colonial Ruling

Globally, colonial interactions had intense and overwhelming social, cultural, political, and economic impacts. Further, gender repeatedly unsettled parochial principles, interactions, customs, and practically in every colonial encounter, the gender ideals of the colonizing powers shaped colonial practices, local laws, and culture. However, these ideals were different depending on the local responses of the colonized people. One example is the US ruling in Hawaii. Before the US control of Hawaii, Hawaiian women played important social, economic, political, and spiritual roles and upheld a significant degree of personal autonomy. However, Hawaiian women were criticized as being sexually immoral and were regularly excluded from US-dominated politics and defined as legally subordinate to Hawaiian and US men, and their legal and social positions were overwhelmingly weakened. However, since the US government allotted Hawaiian land into salable pieces and indigenous people believed that women were better guardians of Hawaiian land, they inherited these lands and became more economically independent. Thus, the apparent impact was safeguarding Hawaiian women's economic and social importance even though their legal status deteriorated due to biased US policies.

Another example is the British colonizers implementing a law in Africa to enforce the idea that wives were the property of their husbands. This was very strange to African gender ideals and permitted men legal control over their wives and being considered the heads of households. Nevertheless, African women used the colonial policies and gained more economic independence through engaging in other occupations like teaching and midwifery. Thus, women with fundamental and critical economic and social roles in their communities were marginalized by colonial policies that visibly preferred men as political and economic actors.

Colonial policies even impacted gender relations in colonialists' home countries. For example, British women started a feminist movement advocating for equal rights to White men and wanted to support Indian women through their superior positions. In this context, British feminists' sense of self as women extensively relied on their knowledge of gender relations in the broader colonial world.

Postcolonial Impact on Colonized Nations

We often think about colonization as an issue or event in the past that has nothing to do with our lives today. However, European colonization had and still has a great deal of influence on many nations, even though Columbus set sail so long ago. These long-lasting consequences of colonization forced nations to deal with many domestic and international challenges to get over the unbalanced and unequal power relationships with past colonizers. To summarize, Europeans started colonizing many nations to gain access to their raw resources to directly enhance their own broken economy. The colonialist system was ruthless in using indigenous people in these nations via slavery, brutality, and death (Campbell *et al.*, 2010). Campbell *et al.* (2010) explain the direct impact of colonialism by asserting that, "[T]he impacts of colonialism were similar, regardless of the specific colonizer: disease; destruction of indigenous social, political, and economic structures; repression; exploitation; land displacement; and land degradation" (p. 37). Nevertheless, colonialism has had lasting domestic and international consequences by creating "artificial states," with an entire infrastructure like roads, rail lines, and lines of communication devoted to the removal of resources from the nation into the hands of the colonizer. Thus, after the colonizers left, "it limited their ability to stabilize their own economy and feed their own population" (Campbell *et al.*, 2010: 37). There were also direct physical effects of colonialism due to domestic political conflicts resulting from independence. This was the case because native people did not influence or know how their own country was run. Thus, the people of the newly independent nation had insufficient information or training on how to run the country (Campbell *et al.*, 2010: 37). Since these nations did not know how to find their place within the international world, it eventually created a vacuum and contributed to the birth of neo-colonialism. Campbell *et al.* (2010) stated that "Neo-colonialism refers to the involvement of more powerful states in the domestic affairs of less powerful ones" (p. 38). It is strengthened by free-trade agreements and development plans that guarantee a company's right to investment above the rights of the citizenry, which means the nation is still abused because of outside meddling disguised as international trade policy.

The Healing Power of Psychotherapy

David and Okazaki, in 2006, created a scale that measures the level of colonial mentality in a person. Their findings are very important because they revealed that people who have higher levels of colonial mentality also had lower self-esteem and higher levels of depression. Fanon (1963), in his groundbreaking research, discusses the colonial mentality as internal oppression created through experiencing external oppression, also known as classic colonialism. The most essential phase of colonial mentality is the "establishment of a society in which the political, social, and economic institutions are designed to maintain the superiority of the colonizer and simultaneously subjugate the colonized" (David, 2008: 120). The colonial mentality is linked to social anxiety, eating disorders, suicidal ideation, substance use, high-risk behaviors, low self-esteem, and depression. Based on this perspective, colonized people highly believe in their own inferiority and behave based on these principles. The most damaging part is that these paradigms are passed down for generations through family systems which maintain these misleading systems of interactional behavior. It is not surprising that research shows a copious number of negative consequences of colonial mentality. David and Okazaki's (2006) research findings account for 62 percent of the variance in Filipino Americans' experience of depression, which is the same for all other groups that have been impacted by colonization.

Internalized Racism as the Consequence of Colonialism

In understanding the impact of colonial mentality, we have to understand and address internalized racism, which is unconsciously embraced by people of color whose countries were colonized. The colonized people moved to the US or other European nations in the hopes of better lives. Still, they get ethni-cally and racially victimized by the same group that took away their resources in their countries of origin in the first place. The most powerful aspect of internalized racism is that people of color develop ideas, beliefs, actions, and behaviors that support or conspire with racism. The systemic reality of internalized racism and the extensive negative consequences for people of color become part of their unconscious reality. Moreover, in the same way that White privilege is part of a system that reinforces the power of White people, there is also a system in place that vigorously dampens and weakens the power of marginalized people and communities of color and drowns them in their own oppression. Communities of color are often unintentionally, consistently, and routinely rewarded for supporting White privilege and power, and they get penalized and rejected when they fail to keep the status quo. This system of oppression is dangerous because it forces people of color to not rely on their own better judgment, weakening the diversity of human wisdom. The same system also deceives communities of color to become adversarial and oppositional through a limited victim/perpetrator lens that decreases the extensive nature of possibilities (Holmes, 2002).

Internalized racism is systemic oppression differing from relational hurts like self-hatred or low self-esteem, which everyone can experience. It is critical to acknowledge its systemic nature and ensure that it is not an individual's problem. It is structural and pervasive and impacts people of color in all aspects of their lives. Therefore, having "high self-esteem" doesn't exempt someone from battling internalized racism, in the same way that the most anti-racist White individuals have to continuously fight their White privilege until this atrocious racist system is eradicated and substituted with a system free of hierarchical racial categories.

It is also important to note that internalized racism negatively influences people of color intra-culturally and cross-culturally due to the horrible histories of dominance and mistreatment. Internalized racism often gets expressed in different cultural and ethnic groups being pitted against each other for the insufficient resources for people without White privilege. This in turn, creates a hierarchy based on closeness to the White norm while it cripples people of color. This often creates great conflict between different minority groups because concepts like ethnicity, culture, nationality, and class are collapsed together, and race is confused with nationality and ethnicity.

If psychotherapy wants to be successful in helping the marginalized and voiceless have a sense of self and agency and become more instrumental in changing their lives, the field needs to challenge the imposition of Euro, cis-male, Christian, and heterocentric norms on psychotherapy. This is the most critical step forward for the psychotherapy profession. The field often talks about multiculturally sensitive psychotherapy. However, the big caveat is that too often, "multicultural" psychotherapy is applied or theorized in ways that in reality perpetuate the same power arrangements they were planning to dismantle. Even though these models were developed to enact and enhance social justice and help marginalized groups, in practice, they get mollified or restructured to fulfill the demands of the same White hegemony they were hoping to counteract and dismantle. In reality, these frameworks are operationalized to reproduce the same existing systems of power and privilege (Vera & Speight, 2003) and continue to colonize instead of decolonizing psychotherapy practices and research. This is more harmful because scholars and practitioners who try so hard to be multiculturally sensitive utilize practices or perspectives that are harmful to the marginalized communities they would like to serve, believing their approach is sensitive and their integrity is intact. Prilleltensky (1997) states an important fact that "discourse without action is dangerous because it creates the impression that progress is taking place when in fact only the words have changed" (p. 530).

Psychotherapy simply cannot concentrate on multiculturalism without a social justice framework because it is deceitful to address the oppression of marginalized people and the oppressiveness of hegemony without paying close attention to the core of their social and cultural experiences. The most tangible way of thinking about this is evident in the very language used to describe, acknowledge, and respond to differences by using words like "cultural competence," "cross-cultural psychology," "multicultural psychotherapy" as if the legacy of inequity and injustice in psychotherapy practices can be centralized only around culture. And that racism, heterosexism, and other forms of oppression are predominantly cultural experiences and are not part of the power dynamics in society or persistent societal arrangements. For example, Aikman (1997) investigated the intercultural education program's conceptualization and application throughout Latin America in the 1980s and 1990s. He noticed that the movement "developed out of concern and respect for indigenous knowledge and practices, but primarily in response to the exploitation, oppression, and discrimination of indigenous peoples" (p. 466). To put it another way, initially, intercultural education would end the colonial educational structures based on a form of cultural genocide by degrading indigenous cultural beliefs and rejecting indigenous experience altogether (Wane, 2008). However, the power system in the country designed the program in a way that rarely jeopardizes the exploitation and oppression of marginalized people to protect the interests of the powerful inside and outside of the country. Another example is related to so many textbooks covering topics related to multicultural psychotherapy teaching therapists how to counsel African Americans, Latinos, or Asians (even though they are not monolithic groups). Nevertheless, this paradigm demands absolutely nothing different from the colonizers. It is not even a remote threat to the prevailing social conditions because it does not challenge the colonizer's sense of power and privilege. It only provides a framework for psychotherapists to distinguish and understand exaggerated group differences from the White "norm." It does not cross-examine or remotely challenge the sociopolitical powers responsible for these cultural injustices. It also does not provide a context for the kinds of systemic oppression, marginalization, and trauma experienced by these groups. This colonial ideology thinking does not even provide a framework outside of dichotomous thinking: white/of color, straight/gay, civilized/uncivilized, Christian/non-Christian, able-bodied/disabled, and binary conceptions of gender (Shirazi, 2011; Leigh, 2009). Instead of strengthening these discourses by providing an analysis of complex systems of power and privilege, these dichotomies maintain the status quo and simply describe the experiences of the disenfranchised people against a hegemonic norm without offering a solution.

Another way scholars and practitioners of "multicultural" psychotherapy have drifted into colonizing ground is by referring to marginalized groups only by the status of their marginalization. Brown (1993) states that these subjugated people are often described as victims and target their oppression. Research about marginalized groups' "struggle for recognition tends to identify the marginalized groups as passive victims" (Li, 2010: 30). The real empowering work should concentrate explicitly on empowering communities of color, communities in poverty, or any other community that has been described as passive and victimized. The biggest contribution of Freire (2000) is the discussion on true liberatory practices that fundamentally reject humanitarian approaches perceiving someone experiencing oppression as a passive object. He advocates for a practice that embraces humanization concentrating on people's own sense of power and agency in their subjective and collective battle for self-determination and liberty. The psychotherapist would ask questions about subordinated cultures through popular multicultural psychotherapy applications in this framework. Psychotherapists must ask themselves how the heteronormative, Eurocentric, patriarchal, and capitalist paradigms influence multicultural psychotherapy. Additionally, psychotherapists need to understand how multicultural psychotherapy practices are strained through the hierarchical and colonizing values dominating psychotherapy practices. González (2003) calls this the "illusion of a free exchange of ideas" (p. 184), even though they clearly subordinate marginalized people and their experiences.

If we want to have a decolonial or postcolonial stance, we need to be concerned about marginalized people's access to power and opportunities (Hernandez-Wolfe, 2011). A decolonizing stance should challenge psychotherapists to stare straight at the power hierarchy, where discriminations are entrenched in systems and organizations that privilege the few at the expense of the many. Shome and Hegde (2002) assert that "the postcolonial project's commitment and goals are interventionist and highly political. In its best work, it theorizes not just colonial conditions but also theorizes why those conditions are what they are, and how they can be undone and redone" (p. 250). Psychotherapists need to reflect on the kinds of multiculturalism they are practicing and examine who benefits and what we protect.

Signs of Colonial Mentality and its Implications for Clinical Practice

The ongoing influence of colonization has long impacted both White and people of color interacting with each other and our internalized belief systems about the superiority of White people. Further, even though many nations have gained independence from formal colonization, it would be careless to think that colonial mentality, which represents internalized cultural inferiority, is not part of our everyday experiences. Among many others, Edward Said (1978), and Frantz Fanon (1963) have discussed colonial mentality in great detail. It is helpful to mention a few points that can help psychotherapists decolonize their thinking and help clients do the same.

Colorism — One of the major residues of colonial thinking is colorism, with both Whites and nonwhites believing that white skin is the universal ideal. This is not about just superficial admiration of whiter skin tone. It is about treating white-skinned people better globally by giving them more opportunities, allowing them to mistreat darker-skinned people, and have a better sense of self based on no accomplishments other than their skin tone. Psychotherapists should understand the consequences of colorism for both men and women. They must discuss the sense of self in therapy and the impact of colorism on how individuals and families view and perceive themselves and others. It is vital to examine the consequence of colonization on how marginalized people view success and accomplishments. People of color often move to the United States due to a lack of opportunities in their colonized country with no resources to prosper. They strive to work hard to make a living and, in the process, deal with all kinds of discrimination and racial tensions. But they give all the credits to their host country for allowing them to live here. They don't realize that they work for the betterment of this nation and not their own. Psychotherapists can help these families appreciate their own hard work and know that the people of their country are not undeserving or somehow lazy. Their governments are corrupt because they inherited a structural system built to benefit the colonizers, not the indigenous people. If clients feel better about themselves, they develop a better sense of identity, and that impacts how they perceive their challenges and accomplishments without giving credit to white-skinned individuals no matter how they get treated.

Preferred communication in English — Colonialism substantially helped raise English as a global language. The ability to communicate in English and other European languages is a significant marker for success and prosperity for immigrant families moving to the Western hemisphere. Further, since colonizers often identified their own languages as superior, they manufactured a local 'elite' who were also Western-educated and spoke English, perpetuating the inferiority of local languages. In his book, *The Wretched of the Earth*, Fanon (1963) explores this phenomenon and discusses the impact of losing the ability to speak the native language as a sign of colonized mentality. Further, since speaking English without an accent is a sign of assimilation, and people of color often suffer from discrimination because they don't speak English without accents, they are often proud that their children speak English. They are often not concerned with their children not knowing their native language. Psychotherapists have important roles in working with people of color because they can explain to families that without spoken language, the culture dies. Therefore, to decolonize people of color's minds, psychotherapists need to encourage clients to reconnect with their own cultural identity, utilizing their native language and culture.

Europeans in leadership positions – A major and effective scheme of European colonizers was to dominate and control colonized people by making them feel inferior through taking over all leadership roles in their communities and managing all aspects of their lives. Consequently, over time colonized people started believing that they didn't deserve leadership roles in their own nations, which kept them silent and unable to speak up against the authority of White colonizers. In today's global communities, Whites are still making decisions for the people of the entire global community, and leadership roles are overwhelmingly arranged and distributed to Europeans. Thus, these leadership positions have been universally accepted despite being based on the old colonial politics. Psychotherapists need to help clients overcome this inferiority complex. They need to help them understand that even in their personal relationship with their family members, they are still looking for White people's ideas, rules, and guidelines to overcome family conflicts. The majority of founders of psychotherapy have been White men, not because they had higher intellectual abilities and skills or knowledge. They were able to have the White establishment support to publish their work and become famous and well known. Many indigenous healing methods can be helpful alongside psychotherapy and can be utilized to help families.

Possessing imposter syndrome – Imposter syndrome can be simply described as a strong sense of not belonging in a professional or personal space. It can be based on not believing in our own intellectual capacity, economic well-being, or not thinking that we may deserve recognition for our work because of race, ethnicity, or class. It is important to note that historically, one of the best colonizing tactics for oppressing people has been making them believe that they are "less than" their colonizers. If they have been given any opportunities, they should be incredibly grateful. This tactic has worked together with the reality that White or white-passing people occupy most global decision-making spaces, and the dominance of White supremacy globally has perpetuated this perspective. Psychotherapists first need to understand the danger of having someone believe that they don't belong in a space based on their racial and ethnic background. Then, they need to challenge this perspective and allow marginalized people to believe in their own intellectual, emotional, and decision-making abilities so they can develop a better sense of self. Only through an empowering process of therapy can marginalized people see themselves as agents who can make sound decisions, be in charge of their own destiny, and value their own contributions to their success.

Seeking validation from Westerners – We need to bear in mind that the majority of nations have been free of the colonial power structure for only the past few decades. In reality, the majority of people still believe consciously or unconsciously in the power and legitimacy of White supremacy, and the colonial mentality persists in all aspects of their lives. Therefore, they are constantly battling with themselves and others to receive validations and confirmations from westerners, which is the dangerous residue of falsely invented colonial dominance. Psychotherapists, first, need to challenge themselves about their own belief systems. Once they understand why they value Western ideas more than other ideas, they need to explore other ways of thinking that might work better for their clients that are not Western solutions. They need to cultivate safer spaces for their clients and involve themselves in the expressed, integrated anti-oppression and decolonizing practices. They must recognize that since we all have gaps in our awareness, we must engage in an ongoing practice of self-exploration and constant learning processes to decolonize our own minds. Below are a few ideas for psychotherapists to decolonize their own minds and help their clients:

1. There are definite power dynamics in any therapeutic relationship that need to be acknowledged in order to decrease the hierarchical nature of psychotherapy. This can be done by asking permission to discuss session topics and modalities and seeing if the client approves the approach. Additionally, the client's needs and values should be the center of any discussion in the therapy room instead of the psychotherapists' beliefs and perspectives. The more psychotherapists become transparent about their own biases and assumptions and ask for clarifications, the better the clients' growth. It also helps a great deal to empower the clients by asking them if the therapist can do anything differently or educate ourselves further to support the client better.

2. Psychotherapists need to accept and appreciate the limitations of Western psychotherapeutic models with their predominant emphases on the individual and family of origin. They need to acknowledge the impact of culture, society, inherited influences, and special oppressive colonial systems that have impacted 90 percent of the world's population one way or another.

3. There are major differences between cultural competency, decolonizing our mentality, and anti-oppressive skills and techniques. Psychotherapists need to understand clients' cultural systems and learn about the influences of the colonial systems their clients continue to navigate.

4. The best practice model for psychotherapists is learning to become transparent and honest about their own interconnecting identities, opportunities, privileges, and lived experiences to assess the impact on the client's experiences. Then, clients can decide if the therapy room is a safe space for them to explore their pain and suffering without being blamed and judged.

5. Psychotherapists need to be highly critical of the psychological diagnoses and acknowledge that Western psychology frequently and repeatedly pathologizes normal, appropriate responses to devaluation, oppression, and trauma. The most appropriate approach is to see what the client is comfortable with and feels empowered by.

6. The majority of Western psychology models were not created to understand the pain and suffering of marginalized groups, even though the
   wisdom and practices of indigenous people have influenced some.
   Psychotherapists need to show flexibility and grace in utilizing these
   modalities.
7. In systemic thinking, all parts of life are interconnected, and clients are
   highly influenced by these larger societal systems. Psychotherapists need to
   recognize the limitations and constraints of all these systems.
8. Belonging to a community and having support systems are essential for
   human well-being. Psychotherapists should encourage and empower
   clients to practice self-care, become part of a community, and advocate for
   organizations and institutions to care about their well-being.

Conclusion

Colonization has directed and controlled socioeconomic and educational
opportunities and created health disparities globally for many native groups.
It has profoundly impacted gendered relationships as well. Discourses about
racial and ethnic minorities have been full of negative stereotypes. Some of
these stereotypes are about women of color created based on stories circulated
by the media and colonizers about many racial and ethnic minority women
as victims of domestic violence, arranged and forced marriages, and systemic
helplessness. This is often explained by news media based on women of color's
cultural background, meaning women are being oppressed because of their culture. The men oppressing them are characterized as the norm in their culture
and religion (primarily Islam). The media and mainstream cultural representation of the same issues completely differ when reporting domestic violence and
murders committed by White men. The description never represents White
men as part of a group or religion (primarily Christianity). They are portrayed
as individuals who acted impulsively, and something went wrong.

Interestingly enough, the news media coverage concentrates on oppressed
racial and ethnic minority women and portrays White women as liberated.
Most news stories compare these marginalized women directly or indirectly
to White women. Thus, the racial and ethnic minority women are presented
as highly oppressed and victimized by the patriarchal culture, while White
women, given exact opposition to minority women, appear as living in a liberated and emancipated culture. There is a happy and liberated 'us' versus an
oppressed, victimized, and homogenized 'them.' These images and portrayal
create the impression that the racial and ethnic minority population and the
White majority population lives are very different from each other.

Therefore, the decolonized research and practice about physical and mental
healthcare should focus on the destructive consequences of colonization and
confess to the impact of Western institutions' maintenance of dominance over
indigenous groups through well-established social structures. Psychotherapists
need to understand that these institutions and systemic disadvantages impact

minority peoples' sense of autonomy and self-determination, exacerbating feelings of helplessness and hopelessness. Psychotherapists must realize that colonization of the mind fuels the loss of culture, language, and identity. Their main intervention must focus on decolonizing practices. Psychotherapists must have an ongoing process of challenging, perturbing, and interrupting the dominant social structures and dynamics by demanding the right to self-determination. This may mean a collective and shared movement to change and challenge the social context and create a safe environment for a communal and culturally specific therapeutic healing system. The most important aspect of this therapeutic work is for clinicians to reflect on their own cultural experiences to gain empathy and knowledge about others and suspend their worldview to fully connect to clients' experiences. Self-examination, providing safety and stability, thoughtful self-disclosure, and flexibility all promote a constructive therapeutic relationship.

Further, the marginalized communities' frameworks in psychological assessment, case formulation, and treatment are essential. For example, clinicians should ask questions about social and historical determinants that have influenced the client's collective and individual experiences and their impact on their well-being. This framework is beneficial for clients who blame themselves for their negative experiences. Finally, clinicians should only use psychiatric diagnoses as the last resort since they contribute significantly to stigmatization. It is crucial to remember that diagnosis implies that suffering and disease can be intertwined, which is highly contradictory with a decolonizing perspective. Psychotherapists hoping to do meaningful social justice advocacy work interested in decolonization must build relationships within the BIPOC (Black, Indigenes, People of Color) communities and advocate for social and political changes.

It is also critical that psychological practices create a context for understanding the construction of women and men and the problems that significantly impact them. This may mean a descriptive framework that includes the cultural perspective of gender, including psychotherapeutic interventions like feminist therapy. It is equally important to pay close attention to the emotional dimensions of all relationships and how gender impacts all aspects of affinities for Whites and nonwhites. Gender should also be utilized as a category of analysis, which can offer a tool that would help to make power visible in all aspects of our relationships. Further, we need an in-depth analysis of the theoretical foundations, the scholars that get to promote their models, and the curriculum that privileges White-centered professional training.

This is particularly important for the predominantly White students to scrutinize their socialization in the White culture to participate in and benefit from structural racism despite all their good intentions. This is important work that requires passion and commitment and can best be done by psychotherapists interested in social justice who strongly believe in the incredible healing power of psychotherapy.

References

Aikman, S. (1997). Interculturality and intercultural education: A challenge for democracy. *Tradition, Modernity and Post-Modernity in Comparative Education*, 463–479. https://doi.org/10.1007/978-94-011-5202-0_6

Bandeira Jerónimo, M. (2018). Portuguese Colonialism in Africa. *Oxford Research Encyclopedia of African History*. https://doi.org/10.1093/acrefore/9780190277734.013.183.

Blanton, R., Mason, T., & Athow, B. (2001). Colonial style and postcolonial ethnic conflict in Africa. *Journal of Peace Research, 38*(4), 473–491. Retrieved July 13, 2021, from http://www.jstor.org/stable/424898

Brown, Wendy. (1993). Wounded attachments. *Political Theory, 21*(3), 390–410. https://doi.org/10.1177/0090591793021003003

Campbell, P. J., MacKinnon, A., & Stevens, C. R. (2010). *An Introduction to Global Studies*. Oxford: Wiley-Blackwell.

Conklin, A. L. (1998). Colonialism and human rights, a contradiction in terms? The case of France and West Africa, 1895–1914. *The American Historical Review, 103*(2), 419–442. http://doi:10.2307/2649774

Columbia Electronic Encyclopedia. (2013) (6th ed.) New York: Columbia University Press.

David, E. J. R. (2008). A colonial mentality model of depression for Filipino Americans. *Cultural Diversity and Ethnic Minority Psychology, 14*(2), 118–127. https://doi.org/10.1037/1099-9809.14.2.118

David, E. J. R., & Okazaki, S. (2006). Colonial mentality: A review and recommendation for Filipino American psychology. *Cultural Diversity & Ethnic Minority Psychology, 12*(1), 1.

Fanon, F. (1963). *The Wretched of the Earth*. New York: Grove Press. https://www.worldcat.org › wretched-of-the-earth › oclc

Ferrante, J. (2007). *Sociology: A Global Perspective*. Belmont, CA: Wadsworth.

Freire, P. (2000). *Pedagogy of the Oppressed* (trans: M. B. Ramos). New York: Continuum. (Original work published in 1970).

González, M. C. (2003). An ethics for postcolonial ethnography. In R. P. Claire (Ed.), *Expression of Ethnography* (pp. 77–86). Albany, NY: State University of New York Press.

Hernandez-Wolfe, P. (2011). Decolonization and "mental" health: A Mestiza's journey to the borderlands. *Women & Therapy, 34*(3), 293–306.

Holmes, B. A. (2002). *Race and the Cosmos: An Invitation to View the World Differently*. Harrisburg, PA: Trinity Press International.

Kohn, M., & Reddy, K. (2017, August 29). *Colonialism*. The Stanford Encyclopedia of Philosophy. https://plato.stanford.edu/archives/fall2017/entries/colonialism/

Leigh, D. (2009). Colonialism, gender, and the family in North America: For a gendered analysis of Indigenous struggles. *Studies in Ethnicity and Nationalism, 9*(1), 70–88.

Li, H. (2010). From decolonization of alterity to democratic listening. *Social Alternatives, 29*(1), 29–33.

Mani, L. (1987). Contentious traditions: The debate on sati in colonial India. *Cultural Critique*, (7), 119–156. doi:10.2307/1354153

Merriam-Webster. *Colonialism definiton & meaning*. Merriam-Webster https://www.merriam-webster.com/dictionary/colonialism

Prilleltensky, I. (1997). Values, assumptions, and practices: Assessing the moral implications of psychological discourse action. *American Psychologist, 52*(5), 517–535.

Said, E. W. (1978). *Orientalism*. New York: Pantheon Books.

Shirazi, R. (2011). When projects of 'empowerment' don't liberate: Locating agency in a 'postcolonial' peace education. *Journal of Peace Education, 8*(3), 277–294. https://doi.org/10.1080/17400201.2011.621370

Shome, R., & Hegde, R. S. (2002). Postcolonial approaches to communication: Charting the terrain, engaging the intersections. *Communication Theory, 12*(3), 249–270. https://doi.org/10.1111/j.1468-2885.2002.tb00269.x

Vera, E. M., & Speight, S. L. (2003). Multicultural competence, social justice, and counseling psychology: Expanding our roles. *The Counseling Psychologist, 31*(3), 253–272.

Wane, N. N. (2008). Mapping the field of Indigenous knowledges in anti-colonial discourse: a transformative journey in education. *Race Ethnicity and Education, 11*(2), 183–197. https://doi.org/10.1080/13613320600807667

5 Gender and Religion

Introduction

Religion is a global phenomenon, formed out of the expressions of novel interactions of cultures over time. Several eras ago, mapmakers provided maps that desperately distinguished the localities of world religions. There was a red color for Buddhism that tracked areas from Tibet to Japan and China. The Middle East was streaked green to reveal the landscape of Islam. India was painted yellow for Hinduism, Africa was orange, while all over Europe and the Western half Christianity was painted as blue. Light blue was used for Protestant Canada and the United States in some maps and dark blue for Catholic Latin America. It seemed like the differentiation between religions was clearly marked. However, even though certain territories of the world act as a condensed place for specific religious traditions, the world has never been sure about its religious identity. For example, Hindu in India is a dominant religion, but 25 percent of Indians were Muslims before Pakistan came into existence, with 15 percent of the Indian population practicing Islam today. The largest Muslim country on earth is Indonesia, but it is also the center for the rich Hindu culture and has the world's most important ancient Buddhist shrines. China is home to many religions, with most of its population concurrently incorporating Confucian values, Taoist beliefs, and Buddhist worship practices in their everyday life. The same religious dynamics are true for Korea and Japan. Another example is Haitians, who are believed to be 90 percent Roman Catholic and 90 percent followers of Voodoo.

In an age of globalization, there is hardly any part of the world that includes only a distinct strand of traditional religion today. Globalization has changed the speed of cultural interactions. This effortless course of cultural exchange, growth, amalgamation, and adoption has been going on since the beginning of the time that history was recorded. In fact, the same story of a great flood brought on by heavenly rage and a human who built an ark to escape it has been retold in the biblical book of Genesis and retold by the great religious traditions of Judaism, Christianity, and Islam. Another interesting phenomenon linked to several religious traditions is related to a string of prayer beads used by the Roman Catholics. Rosary was borrowed from Muslims in Spain

DOI: 10.4324/9781003088189-6

who were inspired by the prayer beads of Buddhists in Central Asia. But the fundamental idea came from Brahmans in Hindu India, and we don't know who they borrowed this idea from. Further, Christianity picked up many pre-Christian aboriginal European cultural practices. For example, the idea of saints and the festival seasons of Christmas and Easter were borrowed from indigenous Europeans.

Thus, religion has always been global, contrary to their preaching, with very porous borders. Religions have moved, altered, and intermingled with one another around the globe. It is important to note that if religions are the cultural expression of people's sense of crucial importance, it makes sense that these cultural phenomena would move with people to a new place and interact and change over time the same way people change. Furthermore, even though most religious traditions claim that the truth about their religious traditions is solid and unchangeable, it is undeniable that every religion includes immense diversity of ideas and cultural elements collected and assembled from its other neighboring religions.

Further, it has been noted that religious and cultural traditions can alter and change due to the global spread of people. While Sikhs, Jews, and Japanese may preserve and maintain specific and central parts of their tradition in their immigrant communities, it is also very likely that there are changes in the way they practice their religion. For example, Jews had to deal with the issues of acculturation and the core belief of their faith to see if they wanted to allow outsiders to convert to Judaism. Sikhs and Orthodox Jews needed to contemplate whether the Sikhs and Jews are a community that is defined only by ethnicity and delineated by kinship. The way a religious community tries to transact with others and answer these fundamental questions will shape the way religions in the diaspora become global religions.

On the other hand, Islam, Christianity, and Buddhism have always seen their religious traditions as global and unable to be confined to the cultural boundaries of any region. These religious traditions have universal pretenses and global determinations, believing that their spiritual practices, philosophies, and viewpoints are globally applicable and relevant. The most interesting characteristic of the followers of these competing global ideologies is that they consider their beliefs as intellectually greater than the others. Some followers believe that they are the only group deserving of inheriting the Earth.

These transnational and expansionist religions also have geographical and cultural origins. Buddhists idolize Sarnath, the place Buddha first preached. Muslims go on pilgrimage to Mecca, where God disclosed his message to the Prophet Muhammad, and Christians have a particular appreciation for Jerusalem. However, despite the cultural homogeneity they claim to have, each of these traditions is extraordinarily diverse because everyone adapts these fundamental ideas and practices to their own contexts. Therefore, many Buddhisms, Christianities, and Islams surpass an explicit regional declaration. Still, what they have in common is how all religions have treated women. Thus, the status of women in any given society is the consequence of interpreting religious passages and the cultural and institutional setup of religious communities. In the next section, the link between religious practices, the status of women, and gender inequality in global society will be discussed.

Religion and Gender Inequality

Gender inequality which significantly contributes to social inequality is a global phenomenon. It has different impacts in diverse areas of the world. These variances are mainly due to cultural legacies, historical change, geographical situation, and, most importantly, the religious norms that preponderate in society (Norris & Inglehart, 2004). It is essential to clarify that religion is described here as a belief system that impacts political and cultural practices. Religion is also a multifaceted cultural system of values, signs, and activities in societies (Stump, 2008). Furthermore, religion is central to individuals' experiences and highly reinforces cultures and societies' social, economic, and political trends (Stump, 2008). It is even possible to assert that any social, geographic exploration in many world regions requires a much closer look at religion as a central variable than race or ethnicity (Peach, 2006).

Globally, women's status in societies mostly depends on the analysis of religious texts and the cultural, formal, and contextual system of religious communities. The impact of religious rules and roles is complicated and changes with time and space. It is crucial to start with the premise that both men and women benefit from gender equality (Verveer, 2011). Further, gender equality and women's liberation strongly impact the financial, social, and democratic advancement of global societies and tremendously help the growth of human communities. This progression is impacted by established patterns that are influenced by culture and customs that are fundamentally based on religion. It must be evident then that the status of women in religion directly correlates with women's position in society, which is based on sociopolitical and geographic factors.

To explain this further, it seems like two fundamental issues must be discussed: the substantial impact of world religions on gender inequality and the social status of women, and the extent of religions' influence that regulates the status of women as well as the gender inequality in different societies. This is important because gender inequality is always influenced by a country's level of economic development (Dollar and Gatti, 1999; Seguino, 2011). Today, all religions support male social power and authority in societal constructions, while women are persuaded to partake in religious life (Klingorova & Havlicek, 2015). Further, religious norms and biases may reproduce patriarchal values in all the world religions (Seguino, 2011). In all world religions, the role of God is always appropriated to a man. Women have predominantly been valued as mothers, but even then, as a mother to a son with significant religious roles, like in Christianity. In world religions, women are admired for their role as part of domestic life and not particularly in places of worship or in public places. It is, of course, noteworthy to mention that the true status of women in religion is more complex, as, in some religions, some women have attained important positions (Holm, 1994). In all major religions, women's voices are hardly heard because of the patriarchal nature of societies. All world religions are harmonized on the reverence for women and their central role in family life, mainly focusing on the role of women as mothers and wives, but none support and encourage women's liberation and complete equality with men (Holm, 1994). Thus, gender roles are separated and most unbalanced in major world religions. Women's influences on the construction of religious rules and customs are insignificant, even though some women have succeeded in having their normative views acknowledged. There have been men who advocated for more incorporation of women in religious rituals. It is imperative to remember that all world religions accept normative conditionality, signifying that men and women are equal before God. However, practical conditionality implicating the status of women in religious communities in terms of everyday life is the central issue for women in all societies (Holm, 1994). We must remember the absolute heterogeneity of these global classifications of religions like Islam, Judaism, and Hinduism in all these assertions. Therefore, we must avoid any stereotyping in religious affiliation and only discuss patterns in practice.

Further, studies on religions and the status of women have been very andro-centric, with women not being the subject in these studies until recently (King, 1995). Hopkins (2009) examines feminist geographies of religion, but the study disregards women's position in religious norms and traditions. Hopkins's study examined 50 countries to show the link between religion, the status of women, and the connection to gender inequality. The study revealed a relationship between religiosity and gender inequality controlling for the strong influence of economic development on gender inequality. Other studies have demonstrated the same results (Seguino, 2011; Klingorova & Havlicek, 2015). Religion and gender equality are linked together because societies with a higher level of religiosity accept the influence and power of religious authorities, who support and encourage a patriarchal organization of society (Norris & Inglehart, 2004). This perspective assumes that women who follow the teachings of the religion due to their upbringing and social customs are not pursuing a public life and are not interested in discourses on gender equality. It is interesting to know that the same religious institutions are conducive for women in helping them with economic and social distress perpetuating the same cycle of women's inequality (Klingorova & Havlicek, 2015).

Nevertheless, every religious doctrine is different in terms of its approach to the civic contribution of women. In their study, Klingorova & Havlicek (2015) have revealed the specific religious traditions and their influence on gender inequality and have put them in three categories: (a) countries with mainstream populations having a low level of religious affiliation have shown the lowest levels of gender inequality; (b) Christian and Buddhist countries have shown average levels of gender inequality; (c) countries with the highest levels of gender inequality are the ones following the religions of Islam and Hinduism. At the same time, the present study found that secular states, in which patriarchal religious traditions do not dominate the country, have more noticeable women's public presence. For example, their findings reveal that Buddhist states have higher participation of women in economic life; with a slight distinction between men's and women's level of literacy and education, they appear to have more gender equality than the Christian, Muslim, and Hindu societies (Cabezón, 1992; Gross, 1994). Interestingly, compared to other religions, Christianity has not been critiqued as much, even by feminists, even though women's participation in public life has been visibly less than men's (Drury, 1994). It is also noteworthy that gender inequalities have been less observable in Muslim countries than those adhering to Hinduism. These Muslim countries have more women in parliament, and access to education for women is at a higher level. Hinduism's traditional beliefs that promote negation of women's economic independence may contribute significantly to women's status (Sugirtharajah, 1994), even though the equality of men and women in India is part of the constitution. It is apparent that traditions and customs are nevertheless strongly embedded in their society and do not allow for the realistic execution of these laws.

Globalization and the economic crisis worldwide may impact the global community and religious societies. They will ultimately become more accepting of gender equality because the traditional patriarchal arrangements can no longer be sustainable for families. Nevertheless, unless women study religious texts and develop different doctrines and new interpretations, the patriarchal hierarchies won't change. Only through religious expertise and knowledge can women impact religious institutions to undertake transformations more advantageous to women and gender equality (Gross, 1994). The unfortunate truth is that we have witnessed a change in the opposite direction for the past few decades as religious fundamentalism and post-secularism trends have become more prevalent at the global level (Sturm, 2013). No society has been able to achieve unequivocal progress toward gender equality. If societies are to achieve a higher level of gender equality, governments should provide more economic resources and equal access to education, and encourage women to take part in pursuing public offices at all levels of the government. This can be the only way that gender equality can be strengthened to benefit society as a whole.

Gender and Religion Research Studies

The field of religious studies and social sciences have been researching the link between gender and religion as one of the critical categories of interest as an explanatory and historical category (Avishai *et al.*, 2015; Calef, 2009; Joy, 2010). These research studies often portray specific life circumstances of women (very seldom men) in the context of religion. This portrayal often comprises their religious experiences and practices in everyday life and incorporates different levels of a religious order such as cultural, individual, and institutional. Based on this explanation, gender is not portrayed as a theoretical tool for sociological analysis: it is utilized as a pragmatic, observed, and essentialist classification

(Joy, 2010; Woodhead, 2007). This theory of gender explains the fates of a distinct group of religious women that are perceived as homogenous and their religiosity as biological as opposed to patterns of the practices breeding specific gender rules irrespective of the structural sex. In this view, gender is conceptualized as an abstract classification beyond the real experiences of these social actors with a real sense of identity embedded in institutions and having concrete structural dimensions. However, there is also an emergent awareness in the analysis of gender closely linked with the concept of agency (Avishai *et al.*, 2015). Based on this perspective, women's higher level of religiosity has been linked to their exclusion from the religious power structure. It is understood as subversive or transgressive behavior, offsetting their experience of marginalization and inequality and their lack of formal power. Ironically, these gendered religious practices, inertly or not, serve as means and tools for changing or recreating religious commands. Further, studies on the relationship between gender and religion have been more general and descriptive even when they have used analytical and abstract categories. One tactic to classify the current research is to analyze religion at the micro, meso, and macro level. According to Leszczyńska and Zielińska (2016), research studies should pay attention to individual experiences in religious orders at the micro level, the institutional level at the meso level, or cultural and structural frameworks at macro level, even though these categories are also intertwined and dynamic in social reality. This chapter examines the status of Muslim women in more recent studies. The reason is that for centuries Muslim women have been portrayed as the most oppressed by the patriarchal system in Islam; their head cover has been the center of controversy for many decades, and their gendered experiences have been the subject of numerous studies. The hope is to show the complexity of how gender and religious perspectives are intertwined and how other contextual and ecological factors can impact women's lives, and how women in one religious tradition are fighting for gender equality.

Women In Muslim Societies

Out of almost four billion women, more than half a billion are Muslim, mostly concentrated in nearly 45 Muslim-majority countries. The most significant number of Muslim women live in the South Asian subcontinent, with Indonesia being the most populous single Muslim-majority nation. For a long time, a monolithic categorization of Muslim women and their life experiences in the West has existed, which is misleading about the massive interregional, intraregional, socioeconomic, and class differences in their contexts and position. While there are numerous studies about Muslim women, the Western understanding of Muslim women is unjustifiably impacted by data from the Middle East and North Africa, even though less than 20 percent of the world's Muslims reside in this region.

There is a definite patriarchal gender system that contributes a great deal to the lives and experiences of women in Muslim societies. However, the pre-capitalist system that operates in rural areas across a wide strip of lands impacts Muslims and non-Muslims from East Asia to North Africa. This patriarchal operating system is not religion based. Rather, it is based on extended family honoring kinship, male authority, early marriage often resulting in high fertility, strict rules for female behavior that link family honor with female righteousness, and sporadically, polygamous family arrangement. Additionally, in Muslim dominated regions, the gendered experiences organize themselves around women's covering and sex segregations. It seems like the majority of the recent scholarship solely blames Islam as the leading cause of the positions and conditions of Muslim women without looking more into contributing factors such as the economic structures and strategies or differences in the established cultural customs and value patterns of each region.

Further, the revered scripts belonging to Islam, like those of the other Abrahamic religions like Christianity and Judaism, have been inferred to support patriarchal social relations. However, in recent years, Western researchers have started to look at other religions and the status of women and not portray Islam as exclusively patriarchal and incompatible with women's equality. Most scholars now perceive Islam as no more fundamentally misogynist than other main monotheistic traditions. Finally, most scholars must come to understand that many cultural practices that are oppressive to women and linked to Islam as a religion, such as female circumcision, polygamy, early marriage, and honor killings, are either geographically explicit or far from being the norm for Muslim families.

In terms of family law and its actual execution, Muslim women are often formally encouraged to use rules and policies embedded in the religion to avoid inequitable requirements in the law. For example, women in most Middle Eastern countries can add sections into marriage contracts that make drug addictions, taking another wife, or not paying for all the living expenses grounds for divorce and the division of marital assets after divorce. Therefore, based on the legal systems' limitations to equality, Muslim women have fought to improve many parts of their lives throughout all territories. For example, Muslim women have significantly reduced gender gaps in their societies in education and health. They have made significant achievements in reducing the gender gap between Muslim and non-Muslim societies. Only a generation ago, women in the Middle Eastern and North African regions' education level was the lowest in the world, and now they have achieved parity with men in that region.

Further, macro level analysis has revealed a fast decline in Muslim and non-Muslim differences concerning reproduction. Muslim women had relatively greater fertility and lower contraception use rates for the past few decades. However, Muslim women are now part of the global trend in decreasing fertility. In some cases, such as in Iran, they have attained below-replacement fertility, and this trend has impacted Iran's economy more than any other country. Thus, it seems like broader social and economic influences supersede the special impact of Islam as a religion and an ideology.

There is also a shift in being part of a nuclear family as opposed to extended and multi-generational household living arrangements. Muslim women are also delaying marriage, and many are not even getting married, which changes the traditional patriarchal family structure dynamics. These trends have strongly impacted how Muslim women are tackling topics such as domestic violence, honor killings, and female circumcision.

One of the challenges for the developing economy of any region is evaluating the levels of formal labor force participation. A high proportion of Muslim women work in the informal economy, even though their involvement in the formal economy Southeast Asia is higher. Muslim women's participation in paid work seems to be related to a specific economic development strategy that requires female labor, not to a religious ideology or cultural beliefs in men being the breadwinners and women being the homemakers. For example, since the Middle East and North African region's economies are oil-based, female labor was not needed. On the other hand, Muslim countries needing to develop and maintain their industrial production, such as Tunisia, Malaysia, or Indonesia, have a very high female labor force participation. Additionally, globalization has created increased economic and job insecurity and created the need for female labor since families cannot sustain themselves with only one breadwinner.

Women have also gained the right to vote and run for office in almost all Muslim-majority states, with only Kuwait and Saudi Arabia not joining. It is imperative to note that women are still not highly present and represented, holding high political offices across the globe. However, it is interesting to know that the number of women in high offices has surpassed the world average in the Middle Eastern and North African regions. Moreover, even though Muslim women's presence in politics has been more or less limited, they are highly active in promoting women's rights. They are politically complex, religiously committed, and promote radicalism in their change demands. It is imperative to consider these complexities to better understand the lives of women in different regions of the world.

The Healing Power of Psychotherapy

Even though religion and gender have been ignored and disregarded in the field of psychotherapy for many decades, they both seem incredibly applicable, even crucial, to discuss in the therapy room, with more psychotherapists having become interested in including these issues (Anderson & Worthen, 1997; Kimball & Knudson-Martin, 2002). According to Berger and Luckmann (1966), our experiences in life are socially created through a series of consistent habits and conduct that drift away from their original meaning over time. Although the religious establishment is socially constructed, people experience it as a continuous entity independent of themselves. The process of socialization helps to legitimize religious institutions for future generations. Thus, the same way family processes impact our emotional reactions, religious establishments become part of our emotional bedrocks, impacting people's behavior and affecting the personal meaning they assign to religion. Therefore, we can become apprehensive and uncomfortable if we think or behave outside these established paradigms. Religion is profoundly entrenched in our cultures and even impacts those not practicing any religion. Research reveals that religious involvement, beliefs, or activities offer crucial social support and directly impact the sense of identity (F, 1994; Levin, 1994; Kimball & Knudson-Martin, 2002). Religion also serves as an excellent tool for socialization and character development for both men and women and the designation of relational responsibilities. These relational features that are part of the religious activities, like collaboration, teamwork, and friendships, are often the central foundation for social support for both men and women (Belle, 1991; Ellison & George, 1994; Ferraro & Koch, 1994; Thompson, 1991; Kimball & Knudson-Martin, 2002).

Religious paradigms also assign significant meanings to some moral issues. For example, people don't usually conform because everyone acts that way in society, but people often comply if it is based on religious beliefs. They believe the intercession is not between the individual and society; it is between the individual and God. Further, religion is a social institution susceptible to cultural formations of gender, and gender paradigms are not protected from religious doctrines. In fact, the religious teachings in Islam, Christianity, and other religions have dictated that husbands shall rule over wives, meaning protecting their wives. However, it has been interpreted mostly by men to indicate that they are the decision-makers and have more power, which has justified detrimental actions such as violence, demeaning behaviors, or undermining or not paying attention to women's thoughts and feelings. At the beginning of this chapter, we discussed how religions have approved and sanctioned the patriarchal system placing men's interests before women and putting women in an inferior position to men. Men have been given the position of leaders, administrators, imams, rabbis, pastors, monks, and preachers, which has resulted in gender roles being viewed from men's perspective and serving their interests. However, it is crucial to mention that many religious teachings have made great strides and progress toward recognizing challenges created by the lack of gender equality and have made notable attempts to include women's voices and become more inclusive in their decision-making.

Nevertheless, gender is an influential phenomenon entrenched in social establishments and organizations that we interact with regularly (Kimmel, 2016). Therefore, family and religion establish a central connection in society; men's and women's roles become distinct and continuously recreated. For example, these intensely rooted constructions of gender are the base for power differences and the way power is maintained between women and men. In conventional everyday interactions, couples collaborate to conceal women's power and men's dependencies masterfully. It is more acceptable for women to utilize less direct, less aggressive, and more manipulating influential approaches than men. The appropriate bases of power are also dissimilar (Knudson-Martin & Mahoney, 1999). The past two decades of research reveals that these power

dynamics and gender-based differences continue regardless of these pervasive principles of egalitarianism between women and men (Ball *et al.*, 1995;
Knudson-Martin & Mahoney, 1998; Walker, 1996; Zvonkovic *et al.*, 1996;
Kimball & Knudson-Martin, 2002). We all know that the majority of cultural
metaphors and meanings are structured around gender, and they are never
impartial. They are more or less reproduced in the historical legacy of male-
centered culture and maintained through our everyday interpersonal relations
and social constructions (Kimmel, 2016). Since the male-centered culture is
so prominent, men's attributes are valued more and prioritized over women's
traits, making women more accountable for relational issues (Zimmerman *et al.*,
2001). Thus, psychotherapists, even when they want to be sympathetic to gender
inequality in the relationship, miss these explicit unfair gender dynamics. This
is because many of these inequalities are so intertwined with everyday lives
that we are not able to recognize them. These socially embedded and often
concealed ways that power differences create a set structure for relationships
often do not allow many issues to be raised in the therapy room. Thus, unintentionally, psychotherapists make more accommodations for the powerful partner
perpetuating the same gender dynamics that are socially and religiously sanctioned (Knudson-Martin & Mahoney, 1999; Kimball & Knudson-Martin,
2002). Psychotherapists must understand and acknowledge that cultural and
religious-based gender power dynamics harm individuals' mental health and
contribute to relational conflicts for couples and families. For example, the idea
that men should be "in charge" and make independent decisions because of
their religion's upbringing forces men to deny their dependency needs. It also
constrains their emotionality and forces them to disregard their inner needs,
which often contributes to self-destructive and harmful behavior that brings
them to the therapy room in the first place (Kimball & Knudson-Martin, 2002).
On the other hand, the majority of women's symptoms of depression, anxiety, chemical dependencies, and eating disorders are directly related to lack of
assertive expressions and anger for living in a society that undervalues women
(Kimball & Knudson-Martin, 2002). Psychotherapists must pay attention to
the fact that distressed couples often suffer from inflexible gender dynamics.
They need to recognize that successful couples are able to have more flexible gender-based interactions and egalitarian relationships, leading to a higher
level of intimacy (Gottman, 1994; Gottman, Coan, Carrere, & Swanson, 1998;
Steil, 1997). Thus, paying attention to gender dynamics and socialization and
the impact of religious teachings are crucial in clinical work with couples and
families. It is extremely important to note that inequality in relationships is so
embedded in our society and religious upbringings that the impact is invisible
to clients, and they do not know enough about it to bring it up in therapy. Thus,
it is the psychotherapists' responsibility to be extremely careful not to unintentionally give preferential advantages to one gender and they must understand
that relational inequities contribute to mental health symptoms. Therefore,
clinical interventions must not inadvertently maintain gender inequality

(Knudson-Martin & Mahoney, 1996; Kimball & Knudson-Martin, 2002). It makes so much sense to discuss power and gender dynamics in the session, externalizing them as part of social and religious doctrine and helping couples work with more flexible relational opportunities.

It is proven now that these ancient gender arrangements with not many conscious discussions or decision-making will continue to impact relationship dynamics unless therapists take an active role and offer more flexible options. Kimball & Knudson-Martin (2002: 154), propose four relational principles to address equality:

(1) Equal status (partners hold and express equal entitlement to goals, wishes, and needs, share low status tasks, have equal power to define the relationship); (2) Mutual accommodation (daily life is organized equally around each partner, no latent, invisible power to which one partner automatically accommodates); (3) Mutual attending (attunement of each partner to the other's needs and interests, responsiveness to the other's state is equally demonstrated); (4) Mutual well-being (the relationship equally supports each partner physically, psychologically, spiritually, and economically).

Psychotherapists must acknowledge that not many couples accomplish these goals, and their decisions nearly always favor the husbands' plans over the wives', even when they are doing shared decision-making (Kimball & Knudson-Martin, 2002). Thus, psychotherapists can challenge religiously oriented individuals who often respond optimistically to requests to consider ideas like "all of God's children" or "all of creation." All religious doctrine encourages men and women to be sympathetic, understanding, and caring toward others and to consider themselves as holy creations deserving love and respect. Thus, paying attention to the spiritual aspects in therapy can help with a more conscious thoughtfulness about issues related to equality and fairness. Psychotherapists can use religious values and practices as a firm foundation in developing gender equality. Many religious institutions are now advocating for gender equality and discussing it in their institutions. It is so vital for psychotherapists to recognize that religious leaders can be trustworthy sources that can help therapists in their quest for encouraging equal status and relational support. However, as was mentioned before, some religious beliefs highly support "pragmatic egalitarianism" that suppresses real egalitarianisms and covertly promotes men's power over women whilst acknowledging equality and fairness (Fox & Murry, 2000; Gallagher & Smith, 1999). These structurally based gender and power differences are frequently intertwined with religious tradition and constrain relational choices. Psychotherapists must continue to be considerate and understanding and willing to discuss religious beliefs without becoming confrontational and even confused about seemingly undisputable beliefs encouraging gender inequality. The main goal should be to enable individuals to remain faithful to their belief system while respecting fairness and equality, which is also part of their religious doctrine. Psychotherapists must distinguish between institutional aspects of religion from the spiritual, which provides a better space for personal choices. It may even make sense to ask individuals to consider using prayers to help bring equality and fairness to their relationships.

Furthermore, to advocate for gender equality for clients and respect their religious values and beliefs, psychotherapists must first acknowledge their own emotional and cultural reactions around issues related to gender and religion. They must think about unconscious and conscious thoughts and behavior that seem natural and God-given. Gender dynamics and what prevents people from seeing others as equal are important issues. Psychotherapists must recognize what concepts and issues add to their anxiety and make them uncomfortable. For instance, I become anxious when clients use religion to justify a lack of consideration and kindness toward their partner. Over time, I had to learn to validate their perspectives first before challenging them. After acknowledging that perhaps this is their understanding of their religious doctrine, I ask them if God wants them to make another human being unhappy and how they plan to justify their behavior if they are in front of God. I often tell clients that I share their belief about God but see their responsibilities toward him differently. For example, I discuss how men can be the head of their households without holding a hierarchical position. We now know that we do not have to agree with the clients' stance when it carries moral significance without creating a space for discussing a different ethical positioning (Doherty, 1995). Psychotherapists need to realize that issues related to gender and religion are always emotionally charged and make the therapist feel apprehensive. It is important not to side-step or become confrontational and assess our own defensiveness about gender and religion-related issues and know that we all are entangled with a patriarchal context in all aspects of our own lives.

Conclusion

Religion is a global phenomenon with religious communities and cultural traditions preserving their porous borders. World religions have immigrated with people believing in them from one land to another, shifting and interacting with their host cultures worldwide. We have seen religious communities of the East and the West changing based on their interactions with their multicultural contexts and responding to social changes and global transformations. Furthermore, the construct of gender and power and how it impacts relationships continues to be part of the discourse about religion. A significant portion of recent research in family studies and social sciences reveals that gender roles are predominantly created through religion, cultural traditions, the ecological context, and social nurture. For the past two decades, for instance, there has been increasing scholarship on women in Muslim societies offering an extraordinary restorative view instead of a colossal categorization of Muslim women as the only oppressed group dominating the field of social science. This new academic literature considers complex national, social, ethnic, and political diversity among Muslim nations instead of blaming Islam as the single factor for women's oppression.

Overall, given the fact that there is an inherent strong connection between gender and religion, separating cultural constructs of gender fosters opportunities for progress and therapeutic healing for both women and men. In some situations, the influential nature of clients' religion may have approved and promoted gender constructs that create and support inequality. Thus, when psychotherapists want to tackle religious issues, they must search for the spiritual and personal instead of challenging the emotionally fused aspects of religion to help their clients grow and change. Psychotherapists need to be aware that discussing topics of religion and gender is highly emotional for clients and therapists, so they need to be grounded and understand the impact of these issues on their own personal lives before they can successfully help clients. They also need to show respect for clients' beliefs while inspiring clients to look into new prospects. They need to engage in a discourse about moral and relational issues that are directly linked with gender inequality. Psychotherapists' personal journey should expand their commitment to validate clients' perspectives and utilize their spiritual beliefs and connections with God to promote healthy and wholesome relational change. We know for a fact that if our identifications with gender dynamics change, families and religious institutions will change accordingly.

References

Anderson, D. A., & Worthen, D. (1997). Exploring a fourth dimension: Spirituality as a resource for the couple therapist. *Journal of Marital and Family Therapy, 23*(1), 2–12.

Avishai, O., Jafar, A., and Rinaldo, R. 2015. A gender lens on religion. *Gender & Society, 29*(1), 5–25.

Ball, F. J., Cowan, P., & Cowan, C. P. (1995). Who's got the power? Gender differences in partners' perceptions of influence during marital problem-solving discussions. *Family Process, 34*(3), 303–321.

Belle, D. (1991). Gender Differences in the Social Moderators of Stress. In *Stress and Coping: An Anthology* (pp. 258–274). New York: Columbia University Press.

Berger, P. L., & Luckmann, T. (1966). *The Social Construction of Reality: A Treatise in the Sociology of Knowledge*. New York: Anchor Books.

Cabezón, J. I. (1992). *Buddhism, Sexuality, and Gender*. New York: Albany State University Press.

Calef, S. (2009). Charting new territory: Religion and "the Gender-Critical Turn." *Journal of Religion & Society, (5)*1.

Doherty, W. (1995). *Soul Searching: Why Psychotherapists Must Promote Moral Responsibility*. New York: Basic Books.

Dollar, D., & Gatti, R. (1999). *Gender Inequality, Income, and Growth: Are Good Times Good for Women?* (Vol. 1). Washington, DC: Development Research Group, The World Bank.

Drury, C. (1994). Christianity. In J. J. Holm & J. Bowker (Eds), *Women in Religion* (pp. 30–54). New York: Continuum.

Ellison, C. (1994). Religion, the Life Stress Paradigm, & the Study of Depression. In J. Levin (Ed.), *Religion in Aging and Health* (pp. 78–121). Thousand Oaks, CA: Sage.

Ellison, C. G., & George, L. K. (1994). Religious involvement, social ties, & social support in a Southeastern community. *Journal for the Scientific Study of Religion, 33*, 46–61.

Ferraro, K. F., & Koch, J. R. (1994). Religion and health among black and white adults. *Journal for the Scientific Study of Religion, 33*, 362–375.

Fox, G. L., & Murry, V. M. (2000). Gender and families: Feminist perspectives and family research. *Journal of Marriage and Family, 62(4)*, 1160–1172.

Gallaher, S. K., & Smith, C. (1999). Symbolic traditionalism and pragmatic egalitarianism: Contemporary evangelicals, families, and gender. *Gender and Society, 13*(2), 211–233.

Gottman, J. (1994). *Why Marriages Succeed or Fail*. New York: Simon & Schuster.

Gottman, J. M., Coan, J., Carrere, S., & Swanson, C. (1998). Predicting marital happiness and stability from newlywed interactions. *Journal of Marriage and the Family, 60*, 5–22.

Gross, R. M. (1994). Buddhism. In J. J. Holm & J. Bowker (Eds), *Women in Religion* (pp. 1–29). New York: Continuum.

Holm, J. (1994). Introduction: raising the issues. In J. J. Holm & J. Bowker (Eds), *Women in Religion* (pp. 12–22). New York: Continuum.

Hopkins, P. E. (2009). Women, men, positionalities and emotion: Doing feminist geographies of religion. *ACME: An International Journal for Critical Geographers, 8*(1), 1–17.

Joy, M. (2010). The impact of gender on religious studies, *Diogenes, 57*(1), 93–102.

Kimball, L. S., & Knudson-Martin, C. (2002). A cultural trinity: Spirituality, religion, and gender in clinical practice. *Journal of Family Psychotherapy, 13*(1–2), 145–166.

Kimmel, M. S. (2016). The *Gendered Society*. New York: Oxford University Press.

King, U. (1995). Gender and the study of religion. In U. King (Ed.), *Religion and Gender* (pp. 1–40). Oxford: Blackwell.

Klingorova, K., & Havlicek, T. (2015). Religion and gender inequality: The status of women in the societies of world religions. *Moravian Geographical Reports, 23*(2): 2–11. DOI: 10.1515/mgr-2015-0006.

Knudson-Martin, C., & Mahoney, A. R. (1996). Gender dilemma and myth in the construction of marital bargains: Issues for marital therapy. *Family Process, 35*(2), 137–153.

Knudson-Martin, C., & Mahoney, A. R. (1998). Language and processes in the construction of equality in new marriages. *Family Relations, 47*, 81–91.

Knudson-Martin, C., & Mahoney, A. R. (1999). Beyond different worlds: A "postgender" approach to relational development. *Family Process, 38*, 325–340.

Levin, J. (1994). Investigating the epidemiological effects of religious experience: Findings, explanations, and barriers. In J. Levin (Ed.), *Religion in Aging and Health* (pp. 78–121). Thousand Oaks, CA: Sage.

Leszczyńska, K., & Zielińska., K. (2016). Gender in religion? Religion in gender? Commentary on theory and research on gender and religion. *Studia Humanisryczne AGH, (15)*3, 7. http://dx.doi.org/10.7494/human.2016.15.3.7

Norris, P., & Inglehart, R. (2004). *Sacred and Secular: Religion and Politics Worldwide*. Cambridge: Cambridge University Press.

Peach, C. (2006). Islam, ethnicity and South Asian religions in the London 2001 census. *Transactions of the Institute of British Geographers, 31*(3): 353–370.

Seguino, S. (2011). Help or hindrance? Religion's impact on gender inequality in attitudes and outcomes. *World Development, 39*(8), 1308–1321.

Steil, J. (1997). *Marital Equality: Its Relationship to the Well-being of Husbands and Wives.* Newbury Park, CA: Sage Publications.

Stump, R.W. (2008). *The Geography of Religion: Faith, Place, and Space.* Lanham, MD: Rowman & Littlefield.

Sturm, T. (2013). The future of religious politics: towards a research and theory agenda. *Area, 45*(2), 134–140.

Sugirtharajah, S. (1994). Hinduism. In J. J. Holm & J. Bowker (Eds), *Women in Religion* (pp. 59–83). New York: Continuum.

Thompson, E. (1991). Beneath the status characteristic: Gender variations in religiousness. *Journal for the Scientific Study of Religion, 30,* 381–394.

Verveer, M. (2011). *The Political and Economic Power of Women.* Center for International Private Enterprise [online]. http://www.state.gov/s/gwi/rls/rem/2011/167142.htm

Walker, A. J. (1996). Couples watching television: Gender, power, and the remote control. *Journal of Marriage and the Family, 58,* 813–824.

Woodhead, Linda. (2007). Gender differences in religious practice and significance. In J. A. Beckford and N. J. Demerath (Eds), *The SAGE Handbook of the Sociology of Religion* (pp. 566–586). Los Angeles: SAGE Publications Ltd.

Zimmerman, T. S., Haddock, S. A., & McGeorge, C. R. (2001). Mars and Venus: Unequal planets. *Journal of Marital and Family Therapy, 27*(1), 55–67.

Zvonkovic, A. M., Greaves, K. M., Schmeige, C. J., & Hall, L. (1996). The marital construction of gender through work and family decisions: A qualitative analysis. *Journal of Marriage and the Family, 58,* 91–100.

6 Gender and Politics

Introduction

Women's and men's involvement in official and unofficial decision-making arrangements differ significantly between nations but are commonly in favor of men. Institutional, cultural, economic, and societal influences constrain women's prospects, opportunities, and capabilities to participate in societal decision-making. One significant marker of gender inequality in societies is women's political representation. Explicitly, the ratio of seats in national parliaments held by women is one of three markers to measure gender equality, women's progress, and liberation. Not only are women underrepresented in the political circle at the national level, but they also are not even represented in decision-making in the private sphere in their villages or their own civil societies. Men very often control positions of power, including religious and community leaders, local politicians, and village elders.

On the other hand, women's representation and governance lean more toward capabilities that are defined as feminine and related to social well-being. These representations and decision-making are often informal and hidden and consequently not significantly valued. If we ever want to develop and strengthen democracy at the regional, national, and international levels, it is vital to safeguard the equal participation of women and men in both official and unofficial decision-making processes. What becomes even more problematic over time is that the lack of representation for women becomes intensified for men and women. It then overlaps with other discrimination types involving different ethnic groups, people with lower socioeconomic status, different religions, disabilities, and sexual orientations.

Women's Participation and Representation

One of the biggest challenges regarding women's representation at the institutional and societal level is the social norms. These norms create a challenging context for women to leave their familial positions inside their homes and join the public space in society. Institutional obstacles with inflexible schedules that do not consider women's roles within their families make their participation

DOI: 10.4324/9781003088189-7

even harder. To make sure women can participate in the political arena at the international level, many countries have created a quota system. However, many have already realized that creating a quota system is not enough. Two primary reasons are, first, even though more women try to participate in decision-making in society, they are primarily a small minority embedded in patriarchal political systems, unable to act on women's concerns no matter how hard they try. Second, women politicians have a hard time identifying and prioritizing women's issues because issues like class, race, religion, socioeconomic status, sexual orientation, and disabilities divide women and prevent them from coming together and concentrating on their issues regardless of their differences. Something that men mastered centuries ago.

Nevertheless, quotas and allocation of positions will influence society's views of women and consequently welcome women's leaderships (Beaman *et al.*, 2009). It is imperative to use the quota system and help women develop skills in leadership to strengthen women's voices so they can serve as leaders in their communities. For example, a study by Beaman *et al.* (2009) utilized data gathered from an Indian village council to reveal that the quota system made it possible for women to win council positions. They showed that if communities are exposed to women leaders, their perceptions of women in leadership positions change, and women's leadership abilities will improve. Therefore, more women will receive more votes, and bias against women's leadership will decrease. Wang (2013) studied the increasing participation of women legislators in Uganda and found that the increase has made a difference in pro-women policies. However, the study revealed that other factors such as the support of men in the parliament and the relationship these parliamentary women had with their community were critical. We must realize that increasing the number of women legislators may not be sufficient to develop more egalitarian policies. There is a great need for an empowering environment for women that requires men's support.

Policy Barriers for Electing Women

All kinds of institutional, socioeconomic, and cultural barriers exclude women's successful involvement and participation in politics from getting on the lists of candidates for election. Cross-culturally, politics is perceived by both men and women as a male territory, where it is challenging for women to contribute and be effective. At best, women possess leadership positions in supporting a male candidate. Sadly, it is apparent that although women have been successful in getting into the political arena, they encounter more challenges than men regardless of their level of experience and professional confidence. Furthermore, even after women hold public offices, they struggle to balance their personal and professional responsibilities because society is not ready to allow women to have a healthy relational and career balance.

Another significant issue women face is that they cannot discuss their interest in women's issues before an election, so as not to alienate male voters.

Therefore, there have to be many women occupying and running for these positions in order to get rid of this vicious cycle. There have been instances where women who run for office have faced intimidation and threats because the patriarchal roles and male hierarchy have been challenged. The Inter-Parliamentary Union in 2008 conducted a survey between 2006 and 2008 on achieving gender equality in national politics. They found four elements that are the most impactful for forming a more gender-sensitive legislature: (1) the governing party's support for women's participation; (2) the work of congressional committees toward this goal; (3) the work of other groups in the parliament supporting women, and (4) the guidelines and policies managing the operation of the parliament.

Strategies to Cultivate Women's Participation

Worldwide, the best estimate suggests that less than 19 percent of nation-wide politicians are women (Kangas *et al.*, 2014). Globally, some explicit strategies have been utilized to increase women's participation, including (a) providing training for women to become candidates for political office; (b) offering to fund or create fundraising opportunities for women running for public office, and (c) having women participate in monitoring elections. Other factors are necessary to get women elected, such as motivating women to participate as voters to get more women elected into office and strengthen democracy. Ballington (2011) has created guidelines for growing women's political empowerment organized by voting period, targeting members of political parties, civil society organizations, and activists interested in gender equality. She has presented 20 case studies about political activities and offers concise and explicit selections for political party restructuring. Based on this report, the most successful approach to expanding women's participation in political parties is restructuring political institutions with specific support for female candidates. Tadros (2011) analyzed data from eight countries, reviewing the prospects and restrictions of all the approaches like quotas and other strategies to help women achieve political power. The study revealed that quotas could only work with a strong positive social transformation influence.

Additionally, the study found that supporting women in their political endeavors needs to be based on continuous support after they get elected and not just pre-election assistance. Further, according to Krook and Norris (2014), strong evidence from many countries reveals that the main barrier for women getting elected to serve their communities and countries instead of being based on social, economic, or cultural influences is purely political. This suggests that using religion and culture as significant barriers to the participation of women is a political move and needs to be challenged by both men and women across the globe.

Women's Contribution to Governance

It is apparent that internationally, women are not represented in executive, and administrative positions at the political or private sphere, not even at the local or community levels. This low level of involvement can be directly linked to societal standards and expectations that command heavy domestic roles. These roles frequently leave women with little time to participate in the political arena. Since men have always been involved in political decision-making, governance and political commitment have been viewed as men's responsibilities. Moreover, all conventional and religious leadership positions are run and dominated by men. This is intensely challenging since men are often called to arbitrate disagreements globally, particularly in intermediate justice-related circumstances. Their decision-making process is often based on gendered discriminatory social practices that constrain women's access to justice at the family, societal, and political levels. Even when women hold leadership positions, they are often at organizations that women run. Nevertheless, even though women are not included in political decision-making, they are frequently informally impacted and have decision-making power in their communities as mothers, teachers, volunteers, advisors, small business owners, and community leaders. Women's soundless and discreet leadership often centers around community service. However, it is vital to formally utilize these governance abilities so women can join the governance circle and gain political power for the betterment of their society. Hoare and Gell (2009), in their edited book *Women's Leadership and Participation: Case studies on learning for action*, discuss important programs and expertise needed for women's involvement from Oxfam GB and its partners (Oxfam is a confederation of 19 independent charitable organizations directing their efforts on the lessening of global poverty, founded in 1942 and led by Oxfam International). The book explains the process of a long-term change by offering practical methods and knowledge needed to create a context for women's involvement in national elections as well as female decision-making and ingenuity in community living.

Women's Contribution to Civil Society

We habitually don't think about the gendered sphere when discussing civil society. One of the primary explanations is that we don't consider women's responsibilities in the household and subsequently disregard the household obligations of women that strongly affect their time and energy to participate outside of their household responsibilities. It is not possible to fathom women's contributions and involvement in civil society without integrating an examination of interconnecting disparities and inequities that impact their lives. Howell (2007) advocates for a framework to understand the gender-based relationships in the civil society based on four dimensions of power/family, civil society, state, and market. He claims that these frameworks are all intertwined and permeated by gender relations. They involve culturally explicit roles, identities, standards, and principles that define men and women as socially distinctive beings. Theorizing gender relations as dynamic and adaptive helps societies free themselves from seeing men and women needing distinct roles and responsibilities and encourages women's participation in shaping civil society. Agarwal (2010) assesses community forest institutions in India and Nepal to examine the influence of growing women's involvement in local decision-making. The results support the broader perspective that women need numerical power in order to be more effective with their civic engagement.

Further, they reveal that even when women have numerical power, their strength is about a third of men. Nonetheless, even though women's larger presence is important, according to this study, it is not sufficient. There are other elements like the individuals' abilities, talents, and qualities of decision-making that can potentially help make their participation and presence more successful.

Women-led Organizations

Women have often channeled their leadership abilities through women's organizations and frequently rallied around women's matters. Cross-culturally, organizations that deal with women's issues and are fighting against patriarchal systems are called women's rights organizations. Even though these organizations can have a substantial impact in many instances, due to lack of funding, competition for these limited resources among women's organizations, and lack of support in society, the extent to which they can impact fundamental change is very restricted. It is even more problematic that women's organizations cannot even work cooperatively due to the lack of sufficient resources that all of them can utilize. Nazneen and Sultan (2010) discuss the work of three Bangladeshi women's organizations that motivated women to negotiate their needs with political parties, government, and their supporters in civil society to obtain their gender justice objectives. The results of their study emphasize the significance of a direct commitment of supporters and helpers and the importance of outlining concerns using nonconflictual approaches. They discussed the utilization of personal connections to access new opportunities for activism, even though it can jeopardize their sustainability due to its informal nature. Furthermore, they reveal how unsuccessful collaborations with political parties can diminish organizations' impact and social power.

Gender-Responsive Budgeting (GRB)

Gender-responsive budgeting (GRB) is based on evidence that government policies, budgeting for different programs, spending decisions, and revenue often impact women and men, girls and boys' lives differently due to their dissimilar and distinctive needs and interests. Gender-responsive budgeting ideas create a context for evaluating the different results for different groups. The intention is not to develop independent resources to tackle gender-related issues but to guarantee that government budgets are allotted reasonably to fulfill the most vital needs of individuals and groups (Budlender & Hewitt, 2002). The awareness about gender-responsive budgeting and a universal awareness about how government budgeting impacts civil society was developed in the 1990s (Budlender, 2005, 2009). It is important to note that gender-responsive budgeting is considered part of advocating for gender equality based on the belief that it leads to more successful public fiscal management. It concentrates not only on the content and the categories for budgeting, but it also focuses on the rudimentary policy procedures and processes. It specifically focuses on the issues related to the policy being comprehensive, transparent, and responsible toward gender-based discrimination. These budgeting initiatives are essential tools for gender-responsive budgeting and gender-sensitive policies that ultimately benefit everyone in society. Gender-responsive budgeting demands a substantial and meaningful change in governmental and policymaking practices to employ a different method for designing and budget implementation. It should require the inclusion of all groups of participants that can prioritize fairness and justice and use an ethic of care in all economically related policies and decision-making. Elson (2006) created a report for the United Nations Development Fund for Women (UNIFEM) based on the approaches of the Convention on the Elimination of All Forms of Discrimination Against Women (CEDAW). The study discusses a framework to assess and analyze budgets based on gender equality. The report states that utilizing a rights-based approach can create important criteria for gender equality in governmental budgets.

Further, gender-responsive budgeting should be utilized by non-governmental institutions, foundations, and private organizations, because incorporating the work of all these groups helps with supporting this important work and maintaining the drive and energy to transform and implement responsible economic policy. The distribution and allocation of government money should be based on research and data on gender-responsive budgeting work that has been done hopefully by the parliament and civil society. This provides a broader objective for transparency, liability, and civic engagement and involvement. The partnership amongst civil society and government can also be successful for fostering support for the execution of gender-responsive budgeting initiatives.

Gender Development, Gender Ideology, and Intersectionality

Over the years, women having a part, or not having any part, in the development progression of their country has been gradually assessed. Yet, women's positions in development have been varied based on the way gender roles have been defined. Interestingly, the basic idea related to the equality of men and women was accepted and documented in the UN Charter in 1945 and the UN Declaration of Human Rights in 1948. However, the main group of developmental organizers did not completely pay attention to women's position in the developmental process based on the idea that if men benefit from these decisions, women will also benefit. Globally and over time, the way women's position has been defined has changed. In the 1950s and 1960s, concerns about women in the developmental process were related to human rights issues. Women were helpless entities that needed protection, and there were suggestions about protecting but not consulting them. For example, the UN Conventions were working on issues like Convention for the Suppression of Traffic in Persons and the Exploitation of the Prostitution of Others (1949); Remuneration for Men and Women Workers for Work of Equal Values (1951); and Convention on the Political Rights of Women (1952). During the 1970s, even though women were still not included in the decision-making, there was a recognition that women could contribute to society in more significant ways regarding population control and food-related issues like preparation and consumption. Thus, 1975 became the 'International Women's Year' that led to the UN Decade for Women. In the 1980s, there were more conversations about the impact of gender roles on families and society, which created an inclination to perceive women as necessary instruments and recipients of services and thus vital for the development process. In 1985, the UN Decade concluded with the involvement of many women across the globe in a conference in Nairobi, causing the adoption of the "Forward-Looking Strategies" (Forward-Looking Strategies, 1985). The theme was equality, development, and peace. The sub-themes were health, education, and employment. The conference discussed the barriers facing women in all these areas and made broad recommendations and tactics for overcoming them. They also made some suggestions to governments for generating better prospects for equality for women at many levels.

Gender development: In an examination of sociological research, Ann Oakley examined the distinction between sex and gender. In her view, there is a difference between sex as biological differences and gender as a socially constructed and culturally determined concept (Oakley, 1972; Howson, 2004). Biological and specific physical conditions such as chromosomes, genitals, hormones, and primary and secondary sex characteristics can help determine male or female sex. Gender development, on the other hand, is based on social and cultural perceptions of male and female attributes and roles. There are, however, substantial but not absolute associations between female sex and the feminine gender and male sex and masculine gender. Gender socialization is based on learned behavior reinforced by parents, teachers, peers, culture, and society, even though there are vast differences in how gender roles are perceived across different cultures.

Oakley (1972) discusses several studies and states:

> Professor George Murdock has surveyed the data for 224 societies (mostly preliterate) and shows that the tendency to segregate the economic

activities in one way or another according to sex is strong. Taking a list of 46 different activities, he suggests that some are more often masculine than feminine and vice versa. For example, lumbering is an exclusively masculine activity in 104 of his societies and exclusively feminine in 6; cooking is exclusively feminine in 158 and exclusively masculine in 5. Hunting, fishing, weapon making, boat building, and mining tend to be masculine while grinding grain and carrying water tend to be feminine. Activities that are less consistently allotted to one sex include preparing the soil, planting, tending, and harvesting the crops, "burden bearing" and body mutilation.

(Oakley, 1972: 128)

She mentions that men can play a significant role in raising children in some cultures.

The Arapesh, for example, consider that the business of bearing and rearing a child belongs to the father and mother equally and disqualifies them for other roles. Men as well as women "make" and "have" babies, and the verb "to bear a child" is used indiscriminately by either a man or a woman. Childbearing is believed to be as debilitating for the man as it is for the woman. The father goes to bed and is described as "having a baby" when the child is born... The Trobriand Islanders are renowned for their ignorance of the father's biological role in reproduction, but they stress the need for the father to share with the mother all tasks involved in bringing up children.

Oakley 1972: 134–135)

Thus, gender is culturally specific, and the biological sex of the individual does not determine it. Furthermore, not only does the construction of gender differ from one culture to another, but it is also so dynamic that it changes over time in the same culture based on sociopolitical and economic influences.

Women play a variety of roles in different societies. The law of the land determines their specific roles, standards dictated by religion, socioeconomic status, cultural beliefs, ethnic background, diligence, and household and community productivity for the country. Women are also typically liable for household work, and caring and raising children, as well as the health of their families. More specifically, they contribute to farming, paid household employment services, as well as production of goods and community services. Nevertheless, there is still a broad gap between the contribution of women to society and their political presence and power. Gender has a great impact on how we perceive women's and men's contributions to society. Women's role and participation in decision-making need to be reexamined if we ever want to be fair about their contributions.

Traditionally, the notions of gender have been introduced based on the Western ideal. In this view, most countries' developmental plans center around the deceptive assumption that the nuclear household maintained by a non-industrious wife reliant on a man is widespread. This has never been true in most parts of the world. In *The Family Among the Australian Aborigines*, Malinowski (1913) wrote:

> A very important point is that the woman's share in labor was of much more vital importance to the maintenance of the household than the man's work ... even the food supply contributed by the women was far more important than the man's share ... food collected by women was the staple food of the native ... economically [the family] is entirely dependent upon women's work. (p. 139)

It seems like globally, we need to consult and understand the needs of women and conduct a gender analysis in the most concrete and sensible way by examining specific policies. On the agricultural front, women can be consulted to suggest ways that their work in farms can become easier, such as, for example, providing better equipment and better-quality seeds. With respect to health projects, allowing women to make choices about their bodies and have access to sanitary water may improve their health a great deal. Thus, regardless of helping women function better in society, governmental and policy development must empower women to accomplish their prevailing roles better. An alternate but balancing method is to contest the status quo and seriously challenge the apparent inequalities between the experiences of men and women in society. These structural and fundamental changes can help alter discriminatory laws, allowing women to have more access to lands and grant decision-making power in society. Developmental projects in different nations should encompass all members of a society to the same degree and based on their individual needs.

Gender ideology: Gender and gender role ideology insinuate a mindset dictating the appropriate roles, privileges, and obligations of women and men in society. They suggest general or specific behaviors in the areas of economics, family, law, politics, as well as society. Most gender ideology paradigms are on a continuum from traditional, conservative to egalitarian, and liberal/feminist. Traditional gender ideas often reinforce a clear distinction between the roles of women and men (emotional versus instrumental). On the other hand, egalitarian ideas typically support equal responsibilities for men and women within the context of family relationships. Gender ideology often reinforces pervasive societal politics legitimizing gender discrimination. For example, Lorber (1994) explains gender ideology as "the justification of gender statuses, particularly, their differential evaluation. The dominant ideology tends to suppress criticism by making these evaluations seem natural" (p. 30). Based on this perspective, gender ideology is not on a continuum ranging from conservative to liberal. It actually supports gender classification approaches that differ for conservatives and liberals.

It is important to note that sociologists started measuring gender ideology as early as the 1930s. Kirkpatrick's 1936 Attitudes Toward Feminism scale is an important development in the field of gender studies. Later on, Carole Beere (1990) reviewed the psychometric properties of most gender ideology instruments developed until 1988. Further, the General Social Survey (GSS) and the National Survey of Families and Households include gender ideology scales. Over the years, the correlations, causes, and effects of individuals' gender ideology have been examined by researchers. Overall, gender and birth cohorts impact gender ideology, with men and earlier cohorts revealing more conservative perspectives. Women who are employed and have a higher level of education showed a decrease in traditional views. More conservative gender ideologies are often positively associated with attending places of worship, fundamentalism, and strict and literal understandings of holy books. It is often negatively correlated to education level, socioeconomic status, parental views on gender dynamics, and labor force participation of other people that are relationally close to them. It seems like men's housework and childcare strongly impact men's liberal views about gender ideology. Cross-cultural research reveals that gender ideology strongly correlates with the representation of women in the political arena. Paxton and Kunovich (2003) examined gender attitudes in 46 countries in 1995 using the World Values Survey. The result revealed that even if we control for political and social organizational factors, a conservative gender ideology is negatively and directly associated with the percentage of women who are members of the national legislature of a country.

Intersectionality in women's lives: The concept of intersectionality signifies that often several forms of discrimination based on gender, race, sexual orientation, disability, and class, overlay and interact with each other to form the way diverse groups of individuals experience discrimination. Thus, when we adopt an intersectional approach to women's experiences, we have to be aware that marginalization and oppression are also based on race, class, and economics. Further, while women's experience of overlapping discrimination is unique, it is not solely the totality of different forms of discrimination.

In the feminist way of thinking, the intersectionality of women's lives must serve as a prescriptive purpose. Feminist intellectuals ought to pay close attention to the intersectional nature of social constructions of gender, race, class, as well as inequality. In this more normative sense, intersectionality should consider the differences among women to make sure that the distinctive viewpoints of marginalized women from different races and classes are not suppressed, discounted, or dominated by the voice and needs of more privileged women. Nevertheless, we have to understand that utilizing the notion of intersectionality does not make the conversion to practice any less complicated. However, it is the only way feminist theory and practice can help women move forward.

Women's Movements/Feminism, Politics and States

The feminist movement can be perceived as a subgroup of the "women's movement" that utilizes feminist discourse and encompasses women's identity based on gendered experiences and strives to represent, improve, and rebel against the subordination of women and gender hierarchies (Weldon *et al.*, 2008). This means there should be demands for choice, self-sufficiency, self-governance, gender equality, equity, and ways to destabilize the constructions that preserve male privilege.

Women's movements and feminism, in many ways, represent defiance to the power and control of governing institutions (Weldon *et al.*, 2008). It is apparent that states and countries are critical places for women's movement accomplishments and can either support or obstruct women's progress and access to resources. Researchers have acknowledged the latest area of government action called feminist policy promoting women's status to challenge gender hierarchies (Weldon *et al.*, 2008). Consequently, policy-centered ideas have gradually shifted the actual feminist movements and feminism in practice to make fundamental changes and improvements in women's lives. According to Weldon *et al.* (2008), women's policy agencies (WPAs), which they describe as "state-based mechanisms charged formally with furthering women's status and gender equality" (p. 244) try to create a global context for women's movements to promote participation, representation, and democracy within the government settings. Weldon (2002) stresses that women's movements and women's policy agencies (WPAs) are conceivable delegates for women's interests, the same way government officials are selected. WPAs are responsible for increasing women's participation in the state because they are inclined to hire women. Hence, through enabling women's representation and involvement, WPAs facilitate the process of gender equality, whether the country is trying to move toward gender equality, struggling to preserve gender equality, or striving to make an already established gender equality be part of their policymaking strategies. It seems like succeeding in intertwining state feminism and policy-making might potentially include achieving some level of state feminism as an essential situation leading to democracy or at least explaining democratic stability (Przeworski *et al.*, 2000). According to Weldon *et al.* (2008), state feminism has five essential dimensions:

1. The presence of a women's policy agency or an agency with a formal remit to improve women's status and promote sex-based equality within the context under study – e.g. local, subnational, national, international, etc.
2. The presence of a women's movement (discourse and actors) within the context under study – e.g. local, subnational, national, international, etc.
3. WPAs include women's movement demands into the state.
4. WPAs include women's movement actors (WMA) in the state.
5. The WPA/WMA interplay produces feminist outcomes.

To complete this secondary level, we set forth the dimensions of "feminist outcomes." There are two, either of which is sufficient to constitute a feminist outcome:

5.1   The WPA/WMA interplay produces feminist political processes.
5.2   The WPA/WMA interplay produces feminist social impacts. (p. 256)

Thus, to represent state feminism, WPAs should be able to direct women's movement requests and demands as part of the state policies in order to have a tangible impact on societal changes. It is important to note that Women's Policy Agency or organization can include any state-based agency, at the national or local government and in many branches of the government such as executive or legal. They can formally be appointed to be accountable for supporting the progression and further development of gender equality. Research indicates that the most crucial shift to including gender equality mainly happened in the 1980s and 1990s (Staudt, 2003; Rai, 2003). It is essential to use the word "women" instead of "gender equality." It is more straightforward and more comprehensive and does not exclude the work on gender equality but adequately focuses on advancing women's status. This is a crucial point because gender equality cannot be easily translated into many languages. Thus, the United Nations uses the word "women" to identify the world's policy changes.

The Healing Power of Psychotherapy

All chapters in the book discuss how psychotherapy in general, regardless of the modality (individuals, couples, families), can heal the wounds of our gendered experiences. However, since the institution of family has provided the groundwork for the mistreatment of women that is profoundly ingrained in societal structure, feminist family therapy, more than any other form of therapy, will be influential in helping clients with their gendered relational experiences. This section provides an overview of the philosophies of feminist therapy needing to be incorporated into family therapy.

The family – within the Western hegemonic ideology, a typical family includes a husband as the primary source of economic support, indicating an instrumental role, and a wife who supports the domestic aspects of family life with raising children and performing household duties indicating an expressive role (Parsons & Bales, 1955). This division in the family resulted from the extensive changes in the nineteenth century by separating work from family life. This was the beginning of the period when being productive was valued based on earning money, and those who did not make money did not have an influential position in society. However, if women happened to work outside the home, their expressive and homemaking role did not change, and they worked way more hours than the employed men or full-time housewives. Based on societal expectations, men had more power and status in marital relationships, and women as a group had less power. Today, even though there have been feminist and women's movements challenging all construction of gender relationships, women are even now being treated differently than men and have less power. Research has revealed that chronic powerlessness is the common predecessor for the exhibition of psychological disorders (Boydell *et al.*, 2020; Baah *et al.*, 2019; Lavie *et al.*, 2018; McEvoy *et al.*, 2017; Kim & Dee, 2017). Marital relationship stereotypically burdens women to let go of employment and their homes to adapt to the demands of family life with men. Research has shown that the spouse who sacrifices or changes priorities the most for the sake of the marital relationship stays committed if for no other reason but out of necessity (Hare-Mustin, 1978). The woman, who perhaps has ended her employment, left her family or her own home, to get married has to rely on her spouse to satisfy her everyday needs.

Moreover, the common and very unconsciously ingrained belief that women will adapt to men's way of life often is the basis for the differences in how men and women experience stressful life events. Researchers have found that women are subjected to a comparatively greater degree of change or uncertainty in their lives as opposed to men, causing recurrent psychosomatic symptoms and mood disorders (Hare-Mustin, 1978). Psychotherapists hardly acknowledge these imbalances in the family. It is very common that the power dynamics in the marital relationship are often ignored or overlooked unless the woman in the relationship has more power. It seems like the over-responsible mother and underfunctioning father have been the most significant contributor to severe psychological difficulty for women. This lack of equal partnership often brings couples to seek psychotherapy. However, psychotherapists rarely try to identify and challenge the lack of equity in the family by discussing how many of the relational issues, especially for women, are linked to their subordinate position and have been sanctioned by the larger society (Hare-Mustin, 1978).

Feminist therapy – this modality is based on the premise that the conventional intrapersonal human behavior theories do not acknowledge the prominence of our social context as the most important base for our relational conduct. It further recognizes that society's sex roles and men's and women's position disadvantage women (Rawlings & Carter, 1977; Sachnoff, 1975). Feminism promotes the idea of flexible and adaptable behavior in relation to others instead of masculine and feminine specific behaviors and traits. Feminist therapy has advocated for women to consciously examine the unfairness of the conventional gender roles and find ways to enrich their personal lives to gain self-esteem and learn to define themselves outside the realm of family. The feminist therapeutic connection and interaction represent these values by focusing on the nonhierarchical relationship between the therapist and the client. Feminist therapy concentrates on separating personal from peripheral and focuses on feminist therapy that is nonsexist and is based on the humanistic philosophy (Hare-Mustin, 1978).

Family therapy – the field of family therapy started to grow in the late 1940s and 1950s. Gregory Bateson, Theodore Lidz, Lyman Wynne, and other theorists in the field of family therapy who were studying patients diagnosed with schizophrenia identified the overinvolved mother as the main reason for the development of the disorder. A while later, when soldiers came back from World War II, women who were actively working outside their homes were encouraged to do the right thing and go back to their original responsibilities as wives, mothers, and homemakers. Parsons and Bales's (1955) ideas related to the instrumental roles of fathers and expressive roles of mothers had a powerful influence on the field of family studies. Researchers and clinicians who were noticing these stereotypical sex roles used these ideas as the required conditions for normal family functioning and effective child-rearing. Later, systems theory and family development research focused on the developmental stages, promoting the idea that the normal developmental process must include universal and healthy steps. Normal calamities in the family developmental process usually happen when a member is added or deleted by birth or death. Thus, family therapists using the systemic as well as developmental process can help families function better.

However, gender equality and fairness have been a big challenge for family therapists and feminists to recognize and criticize the flaws of family therapy. The reason is that, even though systems theory can potentially strive for equality and fairness for family members, family therapists, like other members of society, are influenced by the same preconceptions and intolerances as others in the society. They have not been able to let go of their academic training and the conventional emphasis on men's and women's mental health measures. Bowen's Differentiation of Self Scale (Bowen, 1966) assesses the differentiation level based on masculine traits and devalues feminine characteristics as the lack of differentiation. Bowen's approach is very similar to the Ego Strength Scale of the Minnesota Multiphasic Personality Inventory (MMPI), favoring males' traits by including more masculine than feminine scored items (McAllister & Fernhoff, 1976). What seems to be lost in this assessment is the fact that Bowen disregards the strong impact of women's socialization, urging them to be emotional and intuitive and not rational. Thus, it appears that family therapists advertently or inadvertently have strengthened traditional gender role assignments to maintain the status quo and return families to their "healthy functioning."

Consequently, we see that married women often experience a higher incidence of mental illness. The same is not true for unmarried women, which should make us examine the traditional family structure impacting women's mental health. Thus, it makes sense to think that family therapists have to be highly vigilant and alert to ensure that gender role stereotyping does not impact their work. Family therapists must realize that family therapy as an orientation offers better outlooks for social change that is inaccessible from other therapeutic methods. This is because family therapy relies on generational transmission of patterns for behavior and can reflect on the traditional norms and expectations that parents learn from their own families of origin and desperately try to preserve for their current family. The systems approach to family therapy is highly compatible with feminist therapy in exploring behavior based on economic and social factors. The feminist family therapist can mediate in a variety of ways to alter the repressive effects of fixed and inflexible roles on family functioning. As families increase their level of awareness, they become more attuned to acknowledge the sociocultural demands that preserve and maintain traditional gender roles and pursue ways to unburden themselves from these pressures. Examining family therapy methods based on the feminist viewpoint suggests that family therapy is undeniably the most viable option for fighting against inflexible gender roles. The next section will describe how feminist family therapy can be a useful tool to deal with the politics of family therapy in society.

Feminist Theory of Family Therapy

There is a great need for psychotherapists to recognize the impact of societal norms on family behavior, and feminist family therapy models are the most relevant to accomplish this task. Feminist family therapy strives to see relational conflicts based on women's struggles because the majority of traditional family therapy perspectives are based on the male perspective and do not recognize the dominated and often destitute situation for women in families (Gladding, 2018). This section aims to examine the feminist theory and its utilization for improving mental health and the responsibility of the psychotherapists in the process. As mentioned in previous sections, the feminist theory states that human nature shares so many aspects of their being, distinct from sexual differences, and sociopolitical issues are directly related to how women are treated in society.

The feminist family theory believes that our attentiveness to the harshness of traditional gender roles helps family members, both men, and women, assess their sense of self and develop a healthier self-image (Brown & Root, 2014). Research shows that women's mental health issues are different from men's. For example, there is a higher frequency of depression and anxiety in women compared to men, related to body image, socioeconomic status, sexual and domestic violence, single parenting, political issues related to gender dynamics, and many other factors (Brown & Root, 2014). On the other hand, feminist family therapy considers the mental health challenges for men, such as higher suicide rates and higher prevalence of substance abuse, among many other issues that men suffer from due to societal pressures (Smith *et al.*, 2018). Thus, mental health instabilities related to societal gender role expectations combined with the powerlessness to conform to gender role norms create relational difficulties for both men and women. Psychotherapy can first acknowledge these challenges and then help family members develop a mutually equal relationship based on respect for each other's needs. However, this is not possible if psychotherapists do not challenge families to free themselves from the shackles of societal expectations and revise the traditional gender dynamics.

Feminist psychotherapy relies on all stages of therapy to create awareness and promote change. During the assessment process, psychotherapists must pay attention to underlying issues contributing to individual symptoms that are interconnected with larger societal expectations for men and women. Thus, discussing these contributing factors brings them to the conscious level, which helps the therapist and the client collaborate and work together to process these subconscious patterns of thinking. For instance, one of the most straightforward patterns of interaction in families perpetuated in the therapy session is that male perspectives about what needs to change in the family are unconsciously and instinctively accepted more often than ideas proposed by women. Psychotherapists must be able to help both men and women substitute this way of thinking with a paradigm shift in their perception and solution for their family interactional problems. Thus, new ways of thinking that promote equality and fairness must be done by intentionally challenging the unconscious reactions to conventional and automatic thinking.

The most important aspect of feminist family therapy is the egalitarian view of the psychotherapist and client relationship. Feminist family therapists readily acknowledge the fact that clients are absolute authorities and decision-makers for their own lives. However, psychotherapists can offer tools and expert knowledge to confront and alter the traditional gender role patterns that get families stuck and provide a context for equality, fairness, and, most importantly, acceptance (Gladding, 2018). In this perspective, cultural beliefs are critical to consider, but not in a stereotypical way where the unique perception of individuals is ignored. For example, if a family discusses physical punishment of children as an acceptable method of discipline, feminist therapists can acknowledge that many cultures may sanction their perspective. And then discuss the harm that is done by having children think that when they are bigger and have more power, they can also use physical punishment to discipline others and how that contributes to domestic violence in their adult life.

In summary, feminist family therapy is a collaborative and integrated method focusing on the issues related to gender dynamics as a primary source of conflict in relationships between men and women. It can be extremely useful in helping women distressed by unconscious social forces and burdens in the male-dominated society globally. Further, feminist therapy is utterly valuable for men to help them disrupt and challenge the restrictions enforced by dominant masculine ideology preventing them from discovering their true selves.

Conclusion

Psychotherapy has always interacted with politics – at times to interrogate conventional political views and structures and at other times to support the main political views about mainstream issues (homosexuality, cultural practices, etc.). Psychotherapy is fundamentally political since it must continuously pay close attention to a power dynamic between the therapist and the client. On the other hand, psychotherapy has been continually challenged to avoid taking a political stance and has been condemned for its apolitical position in the middle of many moral crises. So, what should psychotherapists do to stay connected to their own professional principles and deal with political issues of the day? Perhaps we can start by looking at some definitions. Dictionary definition of the word "politics" comprises, among other things, the art or science concerned with winning and holding control over a government. Psychotherapists like David Cooper, who is part of the antipsychiatry movement, describe politics as "the deployment of power in or between social entities" (Cooper 1976: 4). Michel Foucault highly influenced Cooper's views in emphasizing the distribution of power instead of possessing power. Cooper acknowledges the fact that power is the fundamental aspect of any interaction. However, it gets structured and employed in many different ways. Carl Rogers (1978) has an interesting view on the topic of politics as well. He states:

> Politics, in present-day psychological and social usage, has to do with power and control: with the extent to which persons desire, attempt to obtain, possess, share or surrender power and control over others and/or themselves. It has to do with the maneuvers, the strategies and tactics, witting or unwitting, by which such power ... is sought and gained – or shared or relinquished. It has to do with the locus of decision-making power ...[and] with the effects of these decisions and these strategies ... (p. 4).

It seems like psychodynamic and psychoanalytic scholars speak confidently about social and political issues. Marriage and family therapists and social workers also discuss political matters, and their views and perspectives are appreciated because they understand the complexity of human nature. Psychoanalytic thoughts have been imperative, particularly in the twentieth century, to explain the gloomy and vicious side of political reality, even though field psychotherapists in general discuss and take a stance about the political matter in a few instances. Feminists and humanistic therapy have been more open to discussing the politics of capitalism and hierarchy.

On another note, we should wonder if psychotherapy is loyal to left or right-wing perspectives. Barry Richards as cited in Totton (2012) states that psychotherapy: "does not bear with it a stable set of political values, which act as a constant factor in combination with other intellectual elements" (p. 6). However, when psychotherapists take on an explicit political stand, it is very often on the left of the political spectrum. It is important to note that most psychotherapists are very silent and can easily be called apolitical or neutral. This often means that this majority is mostly conservatives classifying themselves as neutral and centered, labeling any attempt to discuss political issues by others as leftist and extreme positions. Generally, not many therapists openly claim that they are conservative. Still, in their practice, they advocate for and believe in the private individual, the nuclear family, the need for the restriction of human behavior, and the smallest involvement of the state. Simultaneously, many psychotherapists, including myself, argue that therapy is, in reality, if it is done right is, a radical political activity. Psychotherapists who think otherwise tend not to understand and appreciate their own profession (Totton, 1997).

References

Agarwal, B. (2010). Does women's proportional strength affect their participation? Governing local forests in South Asia. *World Development, 38*(1), 98–112.

Baah, F. O., Teitelman, A. M., & Riegel, B. (2019) Marginalization: Conceptualizing patient vulnerabilities in the framework of social determinants of health – An integrative review. *Nursing Inquiry, 26*(1), e12268. doi: 10.1111/nin.12268. https://www.ncbi.nlm.nih.gov/pubmed/30488635

Ballington, J. (2011). *Empowering Women for Stronger Political Parties: A Good Practices Guide to Promote Women's Political Participation.* United Nations Development Programme and National Democratic Institute

Beaman, L., Chattopadhyay, R., Duflo, E., Pande, R., & Topalova, P. (2009). Powerful women: Does exposure reduce bias. *The Quarterly Journal of Economics, 124*(4), 1497–1540.

Beere, A. C. (1990). *Gender Roles: A Handbook of Tests and Measures.* New York: Greenwood Press.

Bowen, M. (1966). The use of family theory in clinical practice. *Comprehensive Psychiatry, 7*(5), 345–374.

Boydell, K. M., Bennett, J., Dew, A., Lappin, J., Lenette, C., Ussher, J., Vaughan, P., & Wells, R. (2020). Women and stigma: A protocol for understanding intersections of experience through body mapping. *International Journal of Environmental Research and Public Health, 17*(15), 5432. doi: 10.3390/ijerph17155432

Brown, L. S., & Root, M. P. P. (Eds). (2014). *Diversity and Complexity in Feminist Therapy* (2nd ed.). New York, NY: Routledge.

Budlender, D. (2005). *Expectations Versus Realities in Gender-responsive Budget Initiatives.* Cape Town: UNRISD.

Budlender, D. (2009). *Ten-Country Overview Report: Integrating Gender-Responsive Budgeting into the Aid Effectiveness Agenda.* New York: The United Nations Development Fund for Women. Retrieved, *3*(12), 2014.

Budlender, D., & Hewitt, G. (2002). *Gender Budgets Make More Cents: Country studies and good practice.* London: Commonwealth Secretariat.

Cooper, D. (1976). *The Grammar of Living: An Examination of Political Acts.* Harmondsworth, UK: Penguin.

Elson, D. (2006). *Budgeting for Women's Rights:Monitoring government Budgets for Compliane with CEDAW.* New York: United Nations Development Fund for Women (UNIFEM).

Forward Looking Strategies. (1985). *The Nairobi Forward-looking Strategies for the Advancement of Women.* https://www.un.org/unispal/document/auto-insert-207862/

Gladding, S. (2018). *Family Therapy: History, Theory, and Practice* (6th ed.). New York, Pearson.

Gupta, R. (2015, April 13). *The personal is political: The journey of a feminist slogan.* OpenDemocracy. https://www.opendemocracy.net/en/5050/personal-is-political-journey-of-feminist-slogan/

Hare-Mustin, R. (1978). A feminist approach to family therapy. *Journal of Family Process, 17*, 181–194.

Hoare, J., & Gell, F. (Eds). (2009). *Women's Leadership and Participation: Case studies on learning for action.* Rugby: Oxfam. https://gsdrc.org/go/display&type=Document&id=4276

Howell, J. (2007). Gender and civil society: Time for cross-border dialogue. *Social Politics*, *14*(4), 415–436.

Howson, A. (2004). *The Body in Society: An Introduction*. Cambridge: Polity Press

Kangas, A., Haider, H., Fraser, E., & Browne, E. (Eds) (2014). *Gender: Topic Guide*. Birmingham: GSDRC, University of Birmingham, UK.

Kim, Y., & Dee, V. (2017). Self-care for health in rural Hispanic women at risk for postpartum depression. *Journal of Matern Child Health* Jan;21(1): 77–84. doi: 10.1007/s10995-016-2096-8. PMID: 27435729

Kirkpatrick, C. (1936). The construction of a belief-pattern scale for measuring attitudes toward feminism. *Journal of Social Psychology*, *7*(4), 421–437.

Krook, M. L., & Norris, P. (2014). Beyond quotas: Strategies to promote gender equality in elected office. *Political Studies*, *62*(1), 2–20.

Lavie-Ajayi, M., Moran, G. S., Levav, I., Porat, R., Reches, T., Goldfracht, M., & Gal, G. (2018). Using the capabilities approach to understand inequality in primary health-care services for people with severe mental illness. *Israel Journal of Health Policy Research*, *7*(1), 1–9. doi: 10.1186/s13584-018-0236-x.

Lorber, J. (1994). *Paradoxes of Gender*. New Haven, CT: Yale University Press.

Malinowski, B. (1913). *The Family among the Australian Aborigines: A Sociological Study*. London: University of London Press.

McAllister, A., & Fernhoff, D. (1976). Test on the bias: An experiential assessment of sex bias in the psychological battery. *Division 35 Newsletter, American Psychological Association*, *3*(4), 10–12. https://gsdrc.org/go/display&type=Document&id=4269

McEvoy, P., Williamson, T., Kada, R., Frazer, D., Dhliwayo, C., & Gask, L. (2017). Improving access to mental health care in an Orthodox Jewish community: a critical reflection upon the accommodation of otherness. *BMC Health Services Research*, *17*(1), 1–15.doi: 10.1186/s12913-017-2509-4

Nazneen, S., & Sultan, M. (2010). Reciprocity, distancing, and opportunistic overtures: Women's organisations negotiating legitimacy and space in Bangladesh. *IDS Bulletin*, *41*(2), 70–78.

Oakley, A. (1972). *Sex, Gender and Society*. London: Temple Smith.

Parsons, T., & Bales, R. F. (1955). *Family: Socialization and Interaction Process*. Glencoe, IL: Free Press.

Paxton, P., & Kunovich, S. (2003). Women's political representation: The importance of ideology. *Social Forces*, *82*(1), 87–113.

Przeworski, A., Alvarez, R. M., Alvarez, M. E., Cheibub, J. A., Limongi, F., & Neto, F. P. L. (2000). *Democracy and Development: Political Institutions and Well-being in the World, 1950–1990*. Cambridge: Cambridge University Press.

Rai, S. M. (2003). *Mainstreaming Gender, Democratizing the State: Institutional Mechanisms for the Advancement of Women*. London: Routledge, pp. 15–39.

Rawlings, E. I., & Carter, D. K. (1977). *Psychotherapy for Women*. Springfield, IL: Thomas.

Rogers, C. R. (1978). *Carl Rogers on Personal Power: Inner strength and its revolutionary impact (psychology/self-help)*. London: Constable.

Sachnoff, E. (1975). Toward a definition of feminist therapy. *AWP Newsletter*, 4–5.

Smith, D. T., Mouzen, D. M., & Elliot, M. (2018). Reviewing the assumptions about men's mental health: An exploration of the gender binary. *American Journal of Mental Health*, *12*(1), 78–89. Http://doi: 10.1177/1557988316630953

Staudt, K. (2003). *Gender mainstreaming: conceptual links to institutional machineries* (pp. 40–66). https://gsdrc.org/go/display&type=Document&id=4291

Tadros, M. (2011). "Women engaging politically: Beyond magic bullets and motorways." Pathways Policy Paper, October, Brighton: Pathways of Women's Empowerment.

Totton, N. (1997). *Not Just a Job: Psychotherapy as a Spiritual and political Practice*. In House and Totton (Eds), *Implausible Professions: Arguments for pluralism and autonomy in psychotherapy and counselling* (pp. 129–140). Ross-on-Wye, UK: PCCS Books.

Totton, N. (2012). *Psychotherapy and Politics*. SAGE Publications Ltd. https://dx.doi.org/10.4135/9781446218143

Wang, V. (2013, November). Women changing policy outcomes: Learning from pro-women legislation in the Ugandan parliament. In *Women's Studies International Forum* (Vol. 41, pp. 113–121). Pergamon.

Weldon, S. L. (2002). *Protest, Policy, and the Problem of Violence Against Women: A Cross-National Comparison*. Pittsburgh: University of Pittsburgh Press.

Weldon, S.L., Goertz, G., & Mazur, A. G. (2008). *Politics, Gender, and Concepts: Theory and Methodology*. New York: Cambridge University Press.

7 Gender, Race, and Class

Introduction

Racial categories were created to promote the idea that humankind's physical and behavioral differences are genetically based. However, researchers interested in genetic studies in the later parts of the twentieth century could not find biogenetically dissimilar races. Many state that "race" is a social construct forced on different groups of people after European occupations of indigenous nations began in the fifteenth century. The current meaning of the word race referencing humans started to appear in the seventeenth century, and it has had a diversity of implications in the Western world. The word race has been utilized to classify people predominantly by their physical distinctions. For instance, in the United States, race has officially classified people with shared physical characteristics like skin color, hair texture, facial structures, and eye formation. These classifiable physical features are linked with large geographically disconnected populations and labeled as races. That is how there are categories such as African, European, or Asian races. Even when there are no racial categories that a group of people can fit in, many still ascribe race based on any visible physical features that they are familiar with. For example, groups of people who speak one language like Arabs, or the Latin race, practice one religion like Islam or Judaism, or ethnic groups like Chinese or Spanish get lumped together as one race. Throughout the twentieth century until the present time, Western scientists have tried to classify the human race based on their differences. Still, they have not been able to agree on the number of human races that are entirely distinct from each other. What they have agreed on is the fact that human physical dissimilarities do not follow a racial model. DNA analyses have proven that humans have way more similarities than differences with less than one percent variation (Encyclopedia of Britannica, 2020).

Researchers in the fields of anthropology and history were one of the first groups to reexamine race as a social and cultural construct instead of a biological phenomenon. These racial classifications were developed in the late seventeenth century, when Europeans started colonizing different countries, first separately categorizing Europeans from Africans, Asians, and other groups.

DOI: 10.4324/9781003088189-8

But then, in the nineteenth century, it evolved into a novel means for social division and stratification.

Race a Novel Means for Social Division

In the US and other places around different continents, racial categorizations were cleverly used for dividing different human groups. This was an exclusive, systematic, and essential dogma about human differences based on: (1) all people around the globe belong to biologically separate groups called races, but can only be part of one race; (2) phenotypic qualities or the noticeable physical differences are indicators for racial identity to cover those that may not have all the visible racial elements; (3) different races' personality, sense of morality, character, and intellectual capabilities are distinct; (4) races are not equal to each other based on their moral, intellectual, and physical characters. Some are superior, and some are inferior; (5) the racially specific behavioral and physical characteristics of each race are hereditary and intrinsic and cannot ever be changed; (6) different races should be separated and sanctioned to create their own organizations, customs, and societal norms (Encyclopedia Britannica, 2020). Based on these perspectives, Americans gave an inferior social position to African or Indigenous people in the US and passed laws to protect and reinforce these status differences.

The History of Racial Categories

In the late sixteenth century, race as a form of classification of different groups of humans was first used in the English language. By the eighteenth century, race was extensively used for classifying people who lived in the English colonies, with Europeans being viewed as free people, Indigenous people living in the US being viewed as the group that was dominated, and Africans that were brought there being viewed as slave laborers. This legacy is still part of the US culture today. The racial categories were not always based on physical and phenotypic features, but they were created to separate the English from the "Others." They even viewed the Irish as the "Other" and categorized them as savages, and when they were not able to enslave them, they decided to bring in enslaved people from other nations. Once they forcefully dominated the lands of indigenous people in North America, the settlers established plantations that desperately needed free labor, and slavery of Africans being brought in by ships became the best solution. Thus, the beginning of the enslavement and racialization of Africans.

Further, since white settlers needed justification for enslaving Africans, Christianity was utilized as the best justification for eternal enslavement because Africans were considered nonbelievers, and slavery would be a way to save their souls. Additionally, unlike Indigenous people who died from Old World diseases, Africans were immune to these diseases and had nowhere to run in unfamiliar territory. Consequently, Africans became the ideal enslaved people since they had no legal rights, no options to escape, and as non-Christians needed to be saved.

When Chinese workers migrated to the United States to work on building the railroad, white settlers had to deal with a new group with distinct physical and cultural features. While their labor was desperately needed, the public and politicians were against the immigration of the new "yellow peril" as another inferior race. Thus, Congress in 1882 passed the Chinese Exclusion Act. Still, Anglo-Saxon whites who were English, French, Dutch, German, and Scandinavian were not comfortable considering even other European groups like Italians and Greeks to be white. Eventually, the "white" racial category included whites without an Anglo-Saxon background. Therefore, to justify slavery and mistreatment of the Indigenous and other groups, the so-called scientific writings continued into the twentieth century to amplify the dissimilarity between whites and other groups. Science was used as the means for the differentiation of races, providing confirmation for the inferiority of non-Europeans.

Racial Categorization in Asia, Australia, Africa, and Latin America

While Western Europeans were internally dealing with racial categories putting themselves at the top of the hierarchy, they also colonized what they called the Third World in Asia and Africa and used the same racial categories. Even though many of these groups could not fit onto these arbitrary classifications, European conquerors applied the same racial categories. Thus, when colonizers reached the Indian subcontinent, these categories were used for the racial domination by lighter over darker-skinned peoples who had adapted to the hot, tropical nature they reside in.

India's caste system – India included a large population with various physical features and skin tones based on living in either tropical or semitropical environments and immigrations of other people. The Hindus had a sociocultural system separated into restricted, genetic, and endogamic castes. They were hierarchical and had many features of the racial categories. However, the system was not based on skin color and caste included people with all physical distinctions and was not based on the so-called scientific categorization of some being superior and some being inferior. Castes in the past and present are components of a religious system that assigns different values to different people. After the colonization of India, British anthropologists used research to create mutually beneficial relationships with Indians who were upper class and even defended India's caste system. Even though the caste system is now banned in India, it is still powerfully entrenched in cultural norms.

Race in Asia – The insertion of European theories of race in the nineteenth century had a massive influence on Asia, influencing the entire world. The approach was valued as part of Western expertise and symbolized modernity. The racial categories became a new means for the domination of European colonizers and Asian leaders who used them to justify white colonizers' mistreatments of yellow and brown and high and low-status Asians. Colonizers were obsessed with the concept of race and how they could apply it without a clear definition or consistency of use. In fact, they used different methods of this scientific racism to confirm the low racial status of marginalized domestic groups, suppressing them even more. Further, the progression of Westernization and the existence of US military bases in Asia have considerably impacted the beauty ideals for Asians, with lighter skin being considered more attractive.

Latin America – The construct of race is considerably different in Latin America, where there are different groups of people mixed after European colonization: there are Africans brought to the region as enslaved people that are considered Blacks; European colonists occupying these regions that are white; and the indigenous people that lived in that area before European occupation and are called Indians. Before the European occupation, the indigenous population was very diverse but was rapidly destroyed by European diseases and maltreatment. However, the indigenous groups persisted and continued to be relatively large. Thus, Spanish colonists mainly enslaved indigenous peoples, even though they also enslaved Africans. In Brazil, Cuba, and Colombia, indigenous people died so rapidly that the Portuguese and Spanish colonists had to bring in many enslaved Africans. These genetic and cultural integrations among Europeans, Africans, and indigenous peoples resulted in mixed children. Therefore, a new category of mestizo was used for children that were a mixture of indigenous and European colonizers, and mulatto was used for children that were a mixture of African and European colonizers.

Race in the Postcolonial Period

Many nations gained their independence by the mid-nineteenth century, and those who used enslaved people abolished slavery. By the mid-twentieth century, the biological inferiority of persons of color was also disproven. However, the lingering impact of perceiving whites as superior still impacted all these colonized nations. Many countries persuaded Europeans to immigrate to these regions. Still, other nations glorified and celebrated the existence of multiple groups of people intermingling while also discriminating against their own indigenous peoples. Some intellectuals in these countries promoted the idea that the blending of different groups created a more tolerant society and distanced themselves from racial segregation in the US that continued well into the twenty-first century. However, while positive perceptions about physical and cultural blend continue, strong beliefs about the superiority of white culture and whiteness and the inferiority of black culture and blackness and indigenousness bitterly continue. This means that even though multiculturalism has gained prominence, blacks, and indigenous people are still invisible, and their extreme social, economic, and political marginality remains a huge problem to be resolved.

Race and Human Physical Appearance

Researchers have discussed that race and actual physical appearances in humans have no correlations for many years now. For example, African Americans do not have the same physical characteristics. Some have lighter skins, different color eyes, and lighter hair, and some have darker skins, brown or black eyes, and darker hair. Further, in the US, the customary rule is that anyone with known African heritage should be categorized as Black, called the "one-drop rule." This rule was created to allow those classified as racially "white" to continue to enjoy having pure blood uncontaminated by the blood of the inferior races. Interestingly enough, the same rule has not been applied to other "racial" mixtures, like Asians and Latino even though these children have been discriminated against based on their physical features and cannot pass as white.

Class and Racial Exploitation

As mentioned in previous sections, the origins of racial oppression in the modern world go back to colonialism and the slave trade. The colonial expansion of Europe during the sixteenth through the eighteenth centuries and the consequent "turning of Africa into a warren for the commercial hunting of black skins" (Marx, 1967: 751) facilitated the development of capitalism in Europe and later the United States. The slave labor created a context for the astonishing increase in wealth (Du Bois, 1975). Consequently, capitalism in Europe and later the United States became a reality. During the colonial period, the way the slave system was organized in the southern part of the US created a context for the great American way of life for many years to come. Perlo (1988) states: "It was the southern slave owners who, for the first 80 years of the US independence, were major garners of wealth through the forced labor of these slaves and their children and grandchildren" (p. 85). Slaves were treated inhumanely by their white masters and consequently society in general, making them into a product to be used to expand revenue for the owners. Du Bois (1975) states, "These slaves, could be bought and sold, could move from place to place only with permission, were forbidden to learn to read or write, legally could never hold property or marry" (p. 71). After the Civil War and during the Reconstruction period, and after the implementation of segregation, the previously enslaved people that had no other skills than farming became farm laborers working for the same enslavers and later into manufacturing laborers in the mines and mills, earning little money for their labor. Therefore, during years after liberation, with hard work and perseverance, Blacks barely made it to be part of the working class in the United States. Thus, a shifting dynamic created a class structure with whites moving to the middle and upper class and black becoming the working class. Black intellectuals in this era started examining the intersection of class and race, the direct connection between them, and the mistreatment of blacks even at present. With the development of the class structure impacting blacks as well as other groups in the United States, Du Bois (1975) predicted that with the expansion of capitalism in America, blacks would also get engrossed in class conflict.

Gender, Patriarchy, Class

Globally, capitalism and capitalist societies' developmental progress is based on exploiting labor for private profit. This exploitation is facilitated by the capitalist system using racial and gender oppression. Even though patriarchy and racial oppression have existed and exploited humans way longer than capitalism, since the sixteenth century, capitalist society integrated these two systems of oppression for bigger capitalist profit and domination over the working class.

Patriarchy and the oppression of women seemed to have overlapped with the expansion of social classes. Beginning in the eighteenth century and after, capitalism and capitalist relations of production facilitated the exploitation and oppression of women through cheap labor and domestic work to enhance the accumulation of wealth for the upper class. In agricultural societies, men, women, and even children contributed to making life possible on the farm. However, in industrial societies where women became dependent on men's wages, female subordination to male domination through social relations emerged. In this era, class exploitation emerged where both men and women had to work to make ends meet. It seems apparent that class division has been the central theme from slavery to feudalism, to the industrial system, to the oppression of women.

In summary, patriarchy, racial oppression, and class divisions have created the foundation for exploiting labor in capitalist society. Racial and gender separations have served the needs for more profit and wealth through pay disparities between white and other races and between men and women. The racial and gender divides have provided more capital for the wealthy. The use of divide and concur tactics has maintained the white men's power over society and all resources. When we explore the connection between class, race, and gender, we can then understand the broader exploitation of labor to increase revenues for the capitalists. This exploitation is even crueler when it directly impacts marginalized groups and women. Even though some people from marginalized groups and some women can escape the oppression and benefit from capitalist rules, the working class and women and many workers from marginalized groups are the absolute sufferers of capitalist exploitation. This proves that White men have accumulated wealth and power and will continue to benefit from the exploitations of other groups.

The Healing Power of Psychotherapy

A woman's sense of self can be defined in a multidimensional social environment: socioeconomic class, personal and family history, race, ethnicity, history of immigration, sexual orientation, religious and political affiliations, and mental and physical health. Each of these affiliations creates a distinct sense of self that functions together, influencing all social and relational interactions (Almeida, 1998; Falicov, 1995; Hardy & Laszloffy, 2002; Kliman, 1994; Kliman, & Trimble, 1983; McGoldrick, 1998). This intertwined system is multidimensional, with overlaying parts covering individual and family relationships and the increasingly complex social network, neighborhood, community, nation, and global community (Kliman, 1994, 1988).

Discourses provide the language we use for conveying our thoughts and cultural practices (Hare-Mustin, 1994). Our personal narratives help us distinguish ourselves from others and show our own unique sense of self. However, because we have memberships in different dominant and marginalized groups, our identities are often molded by conflicting narratives. For instance, Lucia is an architect and lesbian mother who emigrated from Mexico. She has class benefits as an architect in one domain of her life. Her life is incompatible with any specific group narratives about being a mother, daughter, Mexican, lesbian, and architect. On the other hand, she is not a white, middle-class, heterosexual mother or a white male architect, which defines her marginalized identity. Each of her identities is significant or not significant in different contexts. Therefore, some parts of her contextualized and represented self are concealed from herself and others at different points in her life.

Further, social establishments like schools, justice, child welfare systems, and the media create the dominant discourse. They respond differently to Lucia if her daughter was addicted to drugs than a white woman under the same circumstances. She is also treated differently if she was an undocumented mother from Panama, a heterosexual working-class Italian American, a professional African American, a wealthy French American, or a working-class lesbian from Mexico. These women's reactions to their circumstances indicate their own social positions and associated cultural, class, and gender narratives about mothering and what it means to have a child with chemical dependency problems.

All groups have intertwining and group-specific prevailing and alternate narratives about their sense of belonging. Dissimilarities between groups often exist as hierarchies and can go from best to worst. Hierarchical views of differences increase when people encounter cultural differences, and it becomes very easy to define the dominated group as "others" (Llerena-Quinn, 2001). These different narratives in people's lives often conflict with each other. For example, when a daughter from an immigrant family decides to pursue a life plan against her father's wish, or when a daughter raised in a non-religious family decides to become a religious fundamentalist or a lesbian, these experiences conflict with each other. Some women function biculturally flowing between two cultures, making conscious decisions about being part of the dominant and non-dominant groups (Bacigalupe, 1998). Some other women completely internalize the dominant narratives about themselves, become very self-critical, and either represent their specific group typecasts or struggle to look and act like the dominant groups.

It is important to realize that social diversity and cultural differences are not about the existence of a group of people (us versus them). Still, it is critical to honor human diversity to continue human existence and welfare (Lierena-Quinn, 2001). Culture is a multidimensional, multicontextual aspect of our shared history, principles, and practices. Culture is dynamically changes and grows. It involves all people within that cultural context but is construed multi-fariously by group relationships between individuals and families (Falicov, 1995).

Culture is infused with disparities when it interacts with power and privi-lege, and the location in the social hierarchy affects the level of privilege and power. This, in turn, strongly impacts the belief system and cultural practices. Family dynamics create different degrees of power and privilege, which are enhanced or diminished by family members' level of power and privilege in other areas. Individuals' interactions with each other are often affected when family members execute their intersecting identities based on their perceived level of privilege or marginalization. For example, Lucia is marginalized by her racial identity, sexual orientation, gender, and immigrant status despite her class privilege. On the other hand, her white partner, Mary, has racial and US-born privileges. Mary's stance on immigration and how they are taking jobs away from the US-born and insisting that Lucia should not speak Spanish in public with their child hurts Lucia's feelings.

On the other hand, Lucia has the class and career privilege to hurt Mary's feelings (she is a dental hygienist) by telling her that she was not competent or motivated enough to become a dentist. Thus, the discourses that dominant groups in society create can triumph over other discourses within the family and strongly impact how family members perceive themselves. Each group con-tinuously creates cultural narratives about their self-identities and intersecting relationships. White families' experience with their ethnic identity, social class, religion, and health significantly differs from working-class experiences with racial and ethnic background, immigration status, and health. The experience of being Mexican, lesbian, and having physical disabilities equally differs. In sum, every time one aspect of identity changes, the entire family experience changes as well.

It is important to note that some aspects of our identities seem to be very static, like race (science contradicts the static nature of the construct of race), even though multiracial relationships can also impact our racial identity. Other identities may change when education helps one family member move up, and chemical dependency, disabilities, and teenage pregnancy may get another family member to push down (Kliman & Madsen, 1999). Coming out as gay, converting to another religion, immigrating to another country, and intermarrying all impact our intersectional identities. The class locations can also vary depending on the community we are part of. A teacher belongs to a working-class in a wealthy upper-class neighborhood, but she is considered middle class in another poor neighborhood. All our identities help shape us, even if we are not conscious about them. However, it is much easier for all of us to notice our marginalized identity and dismiss our privileged identity.

Lucia and Mary feel separately hurt by each other because none of them are conscious of their power and privilege. Some aspects of our identities are always overlooked, especially if we are part of the dominant group, and some dimensions of our identities become prominent.

Further, the way we are experiencing our families and communities is gendered and class-bound (Kliman, 1998). This means that belonging to a social class is different from socioeconomic status, a combination of education and income. Social class is not neutral and objective; it is based on relationships emphasizing how the privileged classes live well at the expense of others' hard work and resilience. Therefore, examining social class is different than reviewing socioeconomic status because upper-class life is always at the cost of other classes (Ehrenreich, 1989). Upper-class women who complain about the glass ceiling and unbalanced familial relationships can have the luxury of doing this because working-class women face backbreaking labor and destitution managing the kitchens, nurseries, and offices of these more privileged women. Anna's physician parents paid for her tuition, wedding, and the down payment for her house mortgage, building the foundation for her success. Now at age 55, she can take multiple family vacations and can easily afford to pay for her grandchildren's extracurricular activities. Maria, the daughter of a widowed janitor, did not see a bright future for herself, got pregnant, did not finish high school, later married and divorced another high school dropout. At age 55, she is dealing with severe arthritis and heart problems. She left her job as a secretary to manage life with her disability paycheck. Despite her illness, she takes care of her grandchildren during the week so her daughter can hold a minimum wage job to support herself and her children. Thus, the class strongly impacts women's life expectancies and their family life cycles challenges (Kliman & Madsen, 1999).

Race structures our gendered experiences and shapes all aspects of our lives by either intensifying or decreasing our privilege or lack thereof. When race is combined with capitalism, colonialism, and sexism, it intensifies marginalized families' vulnerabilities (Boyd-Franklin, 2003; US Bureau of the Census, 2020). Joblessness among young Black and Latino men is highly connected to chemical dependency, imprisonment, and violent death, which in turn impacts poor young Black and Latina women (US Bureau of the Census, 2020). The outstanding and painful impact of slavery is directly responsible for a lower expectation for even middle-class black boys compared to expectations for white boys or girls of any class and race. It creates another layer of issues with black women who are often more educated and are employed at much higher rates than black men (Boyd-Franklin & Franklin, 2001).

Consequently, black women do not have to rely on men for financial support; they are married at a lower rate; and enjoy more gender role flexibility compared to any other racial groups (Boyd-Franklin, 2003). Additionally, in the US, the construct of race has often been used to connect to Black and white races only. This has disregarded the other races and the impact of racism on them. Because race is socially constructed and is sensitive to circumstances and context, it is described very differently in diverse nations and territories. For example, many Latinos/as may identify as white based on their status in their own countries, but they get classified as black or brown if they immigrate to the United States. There is also more respect for multiracial identities in different world regions compared to the US.

Ethnicity and immigration status has a circular relationship with gender. The rate of becoming bicultural, multicultural, or assimilating to the host culture varies for everyone based on generation and gender. Some immigrants continue to remain marginalized in their new homes and hold on to the conventional ideas they learned and practiced in their homeland. The younger generations as well as the therapists being raised in the host culture, may discard some of these ideas. On the other hand, some US-born children whose parents assimilated to the American culture may crave a romanticized traditional family life based on the customs in their country of origin. As was mentioned before, race and skin color can make a big difference in immigrants' experiences. Light-skinned immigrants who often had class privilege in their country of origin can adapt quickly, use well-fitting narratives with the dominant American discourses, and make economic progress.

On the other hand, darker-skinned and poorer countrymates continue to struggle both socially and economically. We have seen this trend with European Jews, Russians, and Irish that were poor in their countries of origin. Still, due to their lighter skin color being accepted as white and after generations of biculturalism, they assimilated and became more economically successful in the US. The same pattern has existed for lightskinned color Asian and Latino immigrants. Language is also a significant aspect of ethnic and cultural identity for immigrants, and lack of language proficiency systematically marginalizes non-English speakers.

Moreover, gender and ethnicity discourses overlap with class, race, and religion in complicated and convoluted ways. Sexism, racism, and classism impact women in culturally marginalized groups differently. For example, in many Latino cultures, the concepts of marianismo help to enhance a woman's status if she endures suffering like the Virgin Mary, which make women make way more sacrifices in their relationships with men (Hines et al., 1999). Once they immigrate to the US, this tolerance of their suppressed status which is combined with the harsh realities of Latinas' cultural marginalization, makes them more economically vulnerable. The same way that the labeling of Jewish mothers as overbearing and controlling or black women as nurturing nurses for white children significantly undermines the intricacy of their complicated experiences. Young women from marginalized ethnic communities often encounter both in-group and dominant group sexism that eroticize and overpower them as the "exotic other" (Comas Diaz & Greene, 1994).

Gays, lesbians, and heterosexuals equally have class positions, are part of racial categories, and must deal with their ethnicities, religious backgrounds, political views, and mental and physical health statuses (Greene, 1994). We all know that sexual orientation is influential if frequently concealed, characteristic of family and community life. Homosexuality, bisexuality, and heterosexuality are viewed differently in diverse cultures (Greene, 1994). In the US, the prevalent cultural narratives only allowing heterosexual couples the right to marry have been only a decade ago publicly examined and supported (Bos, et al.,, 2004). In racial and ethnic communities, homosexuality has been viewed as a "white problem," and lesbians belonging to the communities of color have been encountering dismissal or even more marginalization in their own communities for engaging in a "white" practice of sexuality (Greene, 1994). Interestingly enough, a lesbian couple of color might not ever see themselves having anything in common with whites and feel more connected to heterosexual couples in their own neighborhood where they share class backgrounds.

Discussions and perceptions about gender also differ with physical and mental health and ability. Mothers of color have been called enmeshed and overprotective for caring for disabled children. When working-class parents and children deal with illnesses impacting the poor like asthma, obesity, diabetes, or other chronic diseases, their health issues are not perceived as connected to class and gender. Psychotherapists often call a mother resistant or non-compliant if she is poor and unable to make it to the therapy session after taking two different busses to get to the appointment. A single mother with multiple sclerosis living on government disability has an entirely different experience with her illness than a middle-class married mother who can afford private insurance.

Restoration of Relational Hurts in Psychotherapy

The socially constructed differences between individuals can lead to the abuses of power that unconsciously or consciously hurt others. Psychotherapists, by default, even when they are from marginalized communities, always have more power than those who seek therapy. The psychotherapists' inherent power in the room to enforce value is frequently underrated and distorted. According to Hardy and Laszloffy (2002), everyone is hurt when whites' cultural and social values are used as a norm for all other groups regardless of their social status and positions. They suggest that all parties should feel responsible for restoring and healing the relational hurt when it comes to power. Still, the privileged, which in the therapy room is the psychotherapists, should be more accountable for healing since they are more privileged with higher power status. Hardy and Laszloffy (2002) suggested several steps for healing relational hurts: acknowledgment, validation, apology, and forgiveness (AVAF). Acknowledgment deals with accepting the fact that regardless of the intention, the person in power has hurt another person with less power and is aware of the feelings of the person who is hurt. Validation legitimizes the anguished person's feelings. Apology encompasses being accountable for hurting the other person. Forgiveness happens only when the anguished party has accepted the apology and is ready to move on. If the anguished person is not ready, then the person who hurt the other (psychotherapist) must try to acknowledge, validate, and apologize again until the other person is ready to forgive.

The AVAF model proposes obligations for the privileged person, so the followings are some of the tasks for the psychotherapists:

1. Challenge yourself never to think that all sufferings experiences are equal. There are always power differences between the privileged and subjugated experiences. This is exceptionally challenging when people in positions of power feel marginalized in some aspects of their lives. They carry that pain to other relationships and think they are competing with others over who is more hurt and has a higher victim status.

2. Make a distinction between intent and impact since even inadvertent comments and behavior may harm others. It is always critical to recognize the anguish you have caused others without explaining or even thinking you were misheard. This is important because marginalized people are so frequently wounded and traumatized by both intentional and unintentional "micro-aggressions" (Pierce, 1995) by the privileged. The pain that they are feeling should carry more weight than the intention of the privileged.

3. Challenge your inclination to explain away or disprove the experience of the marginalized clients. For example, assuming that women are overprotective or enmeshed with their children when in reality, that is the only way society allows them to define themselves. Another example is blaming the young black man for unemployment when society does not give him fair and proper chances.

4. You must try to have a "thicker skin" that is necessary to react empathetically to criticism, even anger, from a subjugated individual regardless of your own pain and suffering. This is very difficult, but as a psychotherapist, you must be able to separate your experiences of oppression from your clients, so they don't feel obligated to take care of your pain while they are suffering and rely on you for healing.

5. Give yourself permission to have feelings of repentance and not guilt to motivate you to work on a sense of fairness and social justice. It is essential not to allow guilt to overshadow a sense of remorse so you can feel empowered to take corrective actions. This kind of pain can only help you grow and have a sense of accountability toward others.

6. You must resist wanting to leave the therapeutic relationship if you feel that your client does not appreciate you. Remember staying in the relationship and showing accountability is a source of healing for your clients.

As psychotherapists, we are supposed to be healers and helpers. Our career is about helping clients with their injuries of oppression, marginalization, suppression, mental illness, trauma, and relational struggles. These injuries impact clients deeply and can last for generations (Weingarten, 2003). Psychotherapists must tackle the pain and suffering inflicted by oppression on families by incorporating psychological and social healing in psychotherapy. The following guidelines can help psychotherapists help families with their injuries inflicted by power and subjugation.

1.   Try to understand your social location in life. If you want to fully comprehend someone's social location, you must be able to grasp your own social location. Psychotherapists have multiple social positions, and understanding the history of these social positions and memberships can help them to understand the marginalized groups' experiences. There are interconnections between specific theories and clinical approaches that can help connect clients' stories of subjugations and dominations, which is a lifelong process for psychotherapists.

2.   Try to acquire compassion about marginalized clients' experiences of their various memberships. You must challenge yourself to read about the history of marginalized groups, request consultations from experts in their communities, and find diverse settings to gain more experiences with different populations. It is beneficial to ask thoughtful questions and respectfully learn from clients. They should be considered the only experts about their own experiences, senses, and circumstances. You must avoid asking them to educate you about something that you can gain information about yourself.

3.   Try to consider differences as treasured and essential prospects for learning instead of hierarchies of superior and inferior or creating a group for "us" and "the other." Llerena-Quinn (2001) states that we need cultural as well as eco-diversity.

4.   Try to be a coinvestigator with clients in their lives (Anderson, 1997; White, 1995) by considering multiple reasons and meanings for specific traits, and characteristics, without always relying on the dominant explanations. This involves having respectful curiosity and intentional lack of knowledge about a specific situation (Anderson, 1997). We must pay close attention to what is said and not said in the therapy room.

5.   Culturally attuned psychotherapy requires us to deconstruct our dominant knowledge and pay more attention to cross-cultural misunderstandings. Many psychotherapists often don't understand different cultural discourses and offer altered explanations for an experience. Thus, they assign different values to the individual or family experience and may use an unhelpful privileged position. Try to pay close attention to the language and the narrative used by clients (White, 1995), and take a collaborative stance as much as you can (Anderson, 1997).

6.   Psychotherapy can be the best tool to challenge the dominant narratives or strengthen them. Strive to be a culturally respectful psychotherapist and do everything possible to avoid assigning specific meanings to clients' behavior. Marginalized people, including refugees with a history of trauma and survivors of all circumstances, can be listened to with respect or pathologized and defined as severely mentally ill without looking at

their historical oppression. Psychotherapists habitually insist on the great values of individuation and autonomy when working with families from cultural backgrounds that value devotion and interdependency. They often disapprove of parental expectations to continue having a close relationship with their children and encourage young adults to become independent. A colleague once asked me what to do with a Pakistani family he was working with. Their 27-year-old daughter was depressed after getting a divorce and asked them to call and wake her up in the morning to go to work. He perceived this behavior as utterly unhealthy and insisted that they work on their enmeshed relationship. Bacigalupe (1998) labels this nuisance as a colonial practice of excluding the voices of the colonized. If psychotherapists question their own assumptions about gender, race, and class regularly, they can certainly limit the burden of assigning negative meaning to marginalized people's experiences.

7. Culturally sensitive psychotherapists allow all voices to be heard and all ideas to be respectfully discussed (Kamya & Trimble, 2002). One voice should not dominate the conversation, and multiple ideas should be entertained. Intellectual and emotional reactions should both be valued and cherished by respectful listening and responding. Psychotherapists have to be very sensitive and respectful to gender issues and try to have a balanced perspective taking gender, race, and class issues into consideration in every encounter with clients.

8. Culturally sensitive psychotherapists should be willing to continuously learn from clients, colleagues, supervisees, and interactions with others in society. A very religiously conservative middle-aged woman was referred to me by a colleague because her adopted son told his parents that he was gay. My colleague referred her to me because he was working with her son and did not want to be biased by her perspective. During our first session, she told me her son got into a prestigious law school, and she needed to go back to the workforce to support his education. She needed to take several tests, go through intensive training, and was very anxious about her nervousness getting in the way of succeeding. We worked together for eight sessions, and she learned techniques to lower her anxiety and was able to get the job. Contrary to my colleague's assumption, she never once mentioned being sad or anxious about her son being gay. This experience was a great reminder that culturally sensitive psychotherapy must consider several discourses and continue to treat clients as experts on their own life experiences and honor their priorities, not ours. Psychotherapists of color are pressured to treat families from multicultural backgrounds using the same techniques and modalities. However, we sometimes make way more mistakes treating them the same as when we honor multiple identities and relationship priorities. Not all people of color want to see a psychotherapist from their own cultural group in all circumstances. A Filipino woman whose grandfather sexually abused her may not prefer to work with a Filipino psychotherapist who is also part of her community.

A devout Muslim woman may prefer a conservative Christian psychotherapist over a Muslim psychotherapist if she wants to discuss lack of sexual desires toward her husband. An indigenous and Latina lesbian couple may prefer someone who understands the impact of racism and homophobia and how to help them overcome it than someone focusing on their gender and sexual orientation.

9. Clients should be given the liberty to explore differences and similarities between the psychotherapists and themselves, others in their lives and themselves, and clients and their other family members. It should not be up to the psychotherapist to decide whether the differences are small or big or who is more privileged or marginalized. When psychotherapists have more visible privileges than their clients (i.e., white men from the middle to upper class), earning their trust is fundamental to the therapeutic relationship and clients' progress. This can be done by respecting their clients' cultural, sexual, racial, and class differences without judging or indicating superiority and unearned power.

10. Understanding clients' social context beyond their personal and familial environment is extremely important, adding value to our clinical work. Clients often use stereotypical behavior about their ethnic group to justify their own actions. A Middle Eastern or Latino man may justify being disrespectful, hitting his wife, or being more restrictive with his daughters than his sons as the way things are in his culture. Culturally sensitive psychotherapy requires us first to validate the fact that he thinks these are culturally sanctioned behaviors. The second step is to challenge the notion that all men from his cultural groups behave the same way and look for exceptions. A genogram can help to ask him how many men from his culture have been consistently and continuously hitting their wives. Once we find exceptions, we can ask why these men have not behaved the same way and what contributes to their different behavioral patterns. The next step is to discuss how hitting and restricting others from expressing themselves impacts relationships even when women are silent and do not protest or leave the relationship.

11. Recognizing and discovering the compound and, at times, paradoxical cultural and class chronicles impacting our own relational as well as our clients' relational experiences are vital to impactful psychotherapy and developing the prospects for growth in therapy. Psychotherapists must be prepared to ask questions like:
    • How do you think your situation could have been improved or worsened if you had access to more financial resources?
    • What if you had higher or lower education?
    • How do you think your racial background privileges or disadvantages you in life?
    • Do you think your gender or sexual orientation advances or hinders your ability to navigate the social system?
    • What if you spoke a different language?

- What if you lived in another country or belonged to a different faith?
- How do you think your health influences your life decisions?

12. Psychotherapists must be willing to recognize and admit that all our ideas about ourselves and others are based on personal experiences and not an outside force called "objective truth" (White, 1995). Thus, it is beneficial to question ourselves about how we strive to emotionally and intellectually understand our clients' experiences if we have not experienced them in our own lives. There must be a specific set of reactions to life events. If a client's response to a situation seems overboard or out of proportion, we need to contextualize it and understand it from their perspectives and life experiences. Women often are perceived to have more exaggerated reactions to situations. However, because women hold on to so much anguish and pain, they want to express themselves freely and comfortably once they finally come to therapy. Psychotherapists need to create a safe and non-judgmental space to express their bottled-up emotions related to unfair treatments in many circumstances.

13. Psychotherapists always hold a higher level of power and must be liable and responsible for any potential hurt or emotional pain they cause their clients, regardless of their intentions. That is why "self of the therapist" work before seeing clients is so critical. A colleague was working with an Arab Muslim couple. Because the wife was wearing a hijab, she assumed that her husband had more power, and her depressive symptoms were due to the oppression she was experiencing in the relationship and prematurely challenged the husband. The couple stopped coming to sessions and asked for a referral to see another therapist. She reached out to them and asked why they didn't want to continue working with her. The husband explained that he was not even religious, and his wife was a survivor of childhood sexual abuse and decided years later after they were married to wear hijab. He explained that his wife's depressive symptoms were related to her childhood experiences, and he has been her only source of support. The therapist wrote a letter to the wife and apologized for her mistaken and premature judgment. The couple decided to resume their sessions, and the outcome was very successful and healing for the couple.

Conclusion

Families suffer from the multilevel and multidimensional amalgamation of issues in life. However, unbalanced power and privilege impact the lives of women, working-class, and racial minorities more than white middle- and upper-class men. Culturally sensitive and power and privilege conscious psychotherapy can heal the deep wounds inflicted by life events on marginalized groups. It is important to note that even the therapeutic settings can inflict more pain and suffering by unintentionally mistreating women, racial minorities, and working-class individuals. Psychotherapists must offer the kind of relational healing that is authentic and respectful. They should pay close attention to the differences at all levels shaping all relationships. The individuals who choose to come to therapy have already been hurt by those who hold more power and have more unearned privileges. They deserve to be treated with respect and experience accountability, and the best and safest place must be the therapy room (Hardy & Laszloffy, 2002). When anguish and rage are not perceived and recognized (Weingarten, 2003), clients feel more traumatized and want to retaliate rather than heal their own wounds (Kliman & Llerena-Quinn, 2002). Women, racial minorities, and working-class individuals experience much pain and suffering in the local, regional, and global communities (Botcharova, 2001; Kamya & Trimble, 2002; Kliman & Llerena-Quinn, 2002; Weingarten, 2003). We need to make the therapy room a safe place to experience healing and restorative justice.

References

Almeida, R. V. (Ed.). (1998). Transformations of gender and race: Family and development perspectives [Special issue]. *Journal of Feminist Family Therapy, 10*(1).

Anderson, H. (1997). *Conversation, Language, and Possibilities: A Postmodern Approach to Therapy*. New York: Basic Books.

Bacigalupe, G. (1998). Cross-cultural systemic training and consultation: A postcolonial view. *Journal of Systemic Therapies, 17*(1), 31–44.

Botcharova, O. (2001). Implementation of track two diplomacy: Developing a model of forgiveness. In G. Raymond, S. Helmick, & R. Peterson (Eds.), *Forgiveness and Reconciliation: Religion, Public Policy, and Conflict Transformation* (pp. 279–305). Philadelphia, PA: Templeton Press.

Boyd-Franklin, N. (2003). *Black Families in Therapy: Understanding the African American Experience* (2nd ed.). New York: Guilford Press.

Boyd-Franklin, N., & Franklin, A. J. (2001). *Boys Into Men: Raising our African American Teenage Sons*. New York: Plume.

Bos, H. M. W., van Balen, F., & van den Boom, D. C. (2004). Experience of parenthood, couple relationship, social support, and child-rearing goals in planned lesbian mother families. *Journal of Child Psychology and Psychiatry, 45*, 755–764.

Comas-Dfaz, L., & Greene, B. (Eds.). (1994). *Women of Color: Integrating Ethnic and Gender Identities in Psychotherapy*. New York: Guilford Press.

W. E. B. Du Bois & V. Hamilton. The Writings of W.E.B. Du Bois New York: Thomas Y. Crowell Company.

Ehrenreich, B. (1989). *Fear of Falling: The Inner life of the middle class*. New York: HarperCollins.

Falicov, C. J. (1995). Training to think culturally: A multidimensional comparative framework. *Family Process, 34*(4), 373–388.

Greene, B. (1994). Lesbian women of color: Triple jeopardy. In L. Comas-Diaz & B. Greene (Eds.), *Women of Color: Integrating Ethnic and Gender Identities in Psychotherapy* (pp. 389–427). New York: Guilford Press.

Hardy, K., & Laszloffy, T. (1995). The cultural genogram: Key to training culturally competent family therapists. *Journal of Marital and Family Therapy, 21*(3), 227–238.

Hare-Mustin, R. T. (1994) Discourses in the mirrored room: a postmodern analysis of therapy. *Family Process 33*(1): 19–35. doi: 10.1111/j.1545-5300.1994.00019.x. PMID: 8039565.

Hines, P. M., Garcia Preto, N., McGoldrick, M., Almeida, R., & Weitman, S. (1999). Culture and the family life cycle. In B. Carter & M. McGoldrick (Eds.), *The Expanded Family Life Cycle: Individual, Family, and Social Perspectives* (pp. 69–87). Boston: Allyn & Bacon.

Kamya, H., & Trimble, D. (2002). Response to injury: Toward ethical construction of the other. *Journal of Systemic Therapies, 21*(3: Special issue), 19–29.

Kliman, J. (1994). The interweaving of gender, class, and race in family therapy. In M. P. Mirkin (Ed.), *Women in Context: Toward a Feminist Reconstruction of Psychotherapy* (pp. 25–47). New York: Guilford Press.

Kliman, J. (1998). Social class as a relationship: Implications for family therapy. In M. McGoldrick (Ed.), *Re-visioning Family Therapy: Race, Culture, and Gender in Clinical Practice* (pp. 50–61). New York: Guilford Press.

Kliman, J., & Llerena-Quinn, R. (2002). Dehumanizing and rehumanizing responses to September 11. *Journal of Systemic Therapies, 21*(3: Special issue), 8–18.

Kliman, J., & Madsen, W. (1999). Social class and the family life cycle. In B. Carter & M. McGoldrick (Eds.), *The Expanded Family Life Cycle: Individual, Family, and Social Perspectives* (pp. 88–105). Boston: Allyn & Bacon.

Kliman, J., & Trimble, D. (1983). Network therapy. In B. Wolman & G. Stricker (Eds.), *Handbook of Family and Marital Therapy* (pp. 277–314). New York: Plenum Press.

Llerena-Quinn, R. (2001). How do assumptions of difference and power affect what and how we teach. *American Family Therapy Academy Newsletter, 82*, 22–26.

Marx, Karl. (1967). *Capital.* Vol 1. New York: International Publishers.

McClintock, A. (1995). *Imperial Leather: Race, Gender, and Sexuality in the Colonial Context.* New York: Routledge

McGoldrick, M. (Ed). (1998). *Re-visioning Family Therapy: Race, Culture, and Gender in Clinical Practice.* New York: Guilford Press.

Perlo, V. (1988). *Super Profits and Crisis: Modern US Capitalism.* New York: International Publishers.

Pierce, C. (1995). Stress analogs of racism and sexism: Terrorism, torture, and disaster. In C. Willie, P. Reiker, B. Kramer, & P. Brown (Eds.), *Mental Health, Racism, and Sexism* (pp. 277–293). Pittsburgh, PA: University of Pittsburgh Press.

Race. (2020). In *Britannica Online Encyclopedia.* Retrieved from https://www.britannica.com/print/article/488030

US Bureau of the Census. (2020). *Statistical Abstracts of the United States.* Washington, DC: US Government Printing Office. Retrieved from www.census.gov/ prod/www/ statistical-abstract-us.html

Weingarten, K. (2003). *Common Shock: Witnessing Violence Every Day: How We Are Harmed, How We Can Heal.* New York: Dutton.

White, M. (1995). *Re-authoring Lives: Interviews and Essays.* Vancouver, BC: Dulwich Centre.

8 Gender and War

Introduction

More than 40 war conflicts are currently in full force, and approximately 1 percent of people globally are refugees. More than 80 percent of all refugees inhabit in developing countries with scarce resources, while only four million have successfully sought asylum in Western Europe and the United States. Many wars are related to lack of resources, and therefore, it involves being at war with segments of their own country, which broadly includes the poor and certain ethnic groups. Premeditated massacres, execution, torture, people vanishings, sexual assaults, as well as demolishing the social, economic, and cultural structure of societies are globally impacting men and women differently.

The feminist, critical, constructivist, and poststructuralist approaches are beneficial in analyzing the interconnections between war and gender. Cultural interpretations and gendered rules of dominance can perhaps be the primary explanation based on evidence from biology and anthropology disproving that genetics or male bonding can explain warlike traits in men (Goldstein, 2001). The insignificant male and female differences in size and strength and the minor differences in their intellectual capabilities, their exposure to gender hierarchy, and segregation may be associated with war battles for men. However, it cannot justify the definite distinction of gender roles in warfare. Goldstein (2001) sees cultural structures, sexual domination, and financial control as causes of men becoming warriors. It seems like manliness and masculine character is utilized to have men defeat their hesitancy to go to war and assist in creating an operational and cohesive army.

Contrary to popular belief, men are not instinctively inclined to fight in a war. They have to be pulled into the war. They need to be continually persuaded, regimented, restrained when they are at war, and then continuously compensated and respected after returning from the war. In actuality, worries and war trauma are very prevalent for men. The combatant ideology compels men to tolerate trauma and try their best to gain control of their fears, to declare their manhood. Globally, male rites of passage require trials and experiments that exhibit the courage and fearlessness of military practices. Other combatant abilities, such as physical bravery, perseverance, power, competence, and

DOI: 10.4324/9781003088189-9

dignity, are also part of the global traits of male socialization. Courage, self-restraint, and submission to authority are essential qualities for battling fear and require the repression of feelings and emotions. Being sensitive and compassionate is forbidden in war battles, and shame is important for developing masculine traits. Sadly, women have often shamed men and encouraged them to go into war.

Further, militarized masculinity is part of the nationalist culture. For example, World War I was perceived as rebuilding nations, and World War II was perceived as rebuilding Germany (Goldstein, 2001). One of the interesting aspects of war is the expectations from women to motivate, prepare, and send men off to war. Women also represent a safe place to return to and keep things in order for men at war, ironically strengthening the gender order and reinforcing militarized masculinity. Another aspect of this debate is associating women with peace and peace activism which perpetuates the dangerous cycle of perceiving men as warriors and fighters.

Gender as a social construct determines men's and women's relationships based on male domination. The best scientific explanation about men's aggressive and sexually assaultive behavior toward women at war times does not seem to link sexual stimulations with male aggressiveness. Therefore, sexuality and violence are not correlated as the symbolic domination of the enemy's women. Historically, the feminization of enemies has been prevalent across the globe. Thus, men being executed and women being raped and enslaved with their children have been used to feminize defeated people.

Further, sexual assaults and raping women are still widespread even in recent wars. This is due to the continuation of men's woken aggressiveness, diminished social norms, and emasculating the male enemy. This means that by raping women, the conqueror violates the beloved property of the conquered. Metaphorically the victorious groups represent men, and the defeated groups represent women. This may explain the prevalent and extensive homophobia in militaries since gay men are perceived as effeminate, destroying the unanimity needed to conquer a feminized enemy.

Not unexpectedly, even though women now serve in the military in many countries, including the US and the European Union, there is a real struggle against the feminization of armed forces. This is based on the notion that women and peacekeeping have been linked together to challenge battling capabilities since soldiers, by definition, cannot be both combatants and diplomats. This proposition is, to some extent, paradoxical because the United States and the United Kingdom, who are the ones engaging most often in war, also have the highest percentage of women in the force with 14 percent in the US and 11 percent in the UK (Ministry of Defense, 2020; Moore, 2020). Interestingly enough, the issue is not about women being capable of fighting. It is about defending the construction of gender that is linked to masculinity with warfare expertise in defense of femininity. Thus, the military continues to be the best identifier of true masculine identity, and women serving in militaries and having peacekeeping missions weakens the male combatant character.

In sum, the complementarity and parity between female and male armed forces in Europe and the United States that changed the connotations of alliance and protection helps to explain gender as a social construct. Based on this perspective, the construct of gender is an unpredictable classification and has several connotations and different impacts. It strives to shift the discourse about gender beyond the individual level, puts it outside of the gender constructs of warriors, mothers, and lovers, and allows for ways that gender harvests meanings in international security orders. Thus, casting light on gender dynamics is critical and vital for exposing the militarized masculinity that has been persuasively enhanced in constructing the relationship between war and gender.

Gender and War within the Context of the United States

The prominence of male and female status globally has special meaning in understanding war as a gendered experience. During national emergencies such as war, which often jeopardizes the agreed-upon social orders regarding gender, societies have great opportunities to change these hierarchical dynamics. However, historically, new prospects for marginalized groups have been constrained by intense political formations of the implications of war (Encyclopedia.com, 2018). The fictional and traditional definition of war is based on masculine traits and assigns differential duties specified for men and women during wartime. In the US, White men until the late nineteenth century and then all men after that were supposed to safeguard their metaphorical women, homes, and families by serving in the military. Women's presumably passive role as those needing to be protected during war demanded that they preserve these same homes and families, which was assumed to be the best way to support men and anticipate their returns. During American wars, however, the real experiences of men and women contradicts this simple separation because many men did not join the military, and many military men did not serve in a war. Comparably, many women, specifically when the US was at war at home, could access wartime political, economic, and social status that was taken away during peacetime. Still, even within the global cultural context, there has been some flexibility in gendered behavior during wartime, which drastically changes during peace (Gleditsch & Hegre, 1997).

Wartime can have a long-lasting impact on gender dynamics. During the Revolutionary War in the US (Dull, 1985), some women questioned their exclusion from citizenship classifications, categorizing them as the property of free, White, and landowning men. During the same period, free White women started a movement to prohibit imported products, which led to the manufacturing of household items in the US that were so important for the Revolution's victory. The fact that White propertied women were in charge of shopping for home goods put them in the position of decision-making and politicized this movement. The British criticized these women's campaigns to shame nationalist men. However, American White women sustained their progressively more public political activities (Dull, 1985). The same Revolutionary situation helped some northern enslaved African women effectively free themselves and their families (Dull, 1985).

While the Revolutionary and Civil Wars were both domestic wars, the Civil War directly impacted civilians targeted by military ferocity. The attack on civilians mostly happened in the south. Thus, not only did the division between the home front and battlefront become unclear, the distorted correlation between men being protectors and women needing protection really messed up the gender system in the south. Further, the two World Wars of the twentieth century created some fears that assembling a large population to fight the war might destabilize the traditional gender and sexual arrangement. To compensate for this possible risk, during World War II, the federal government created the image of Rosie the Riveter in the media (Gluck,1987). This image portrayed a female worker who, for the first time, entered the labor force to support the war. Rosie the Riveter's image signified a wartime feminine transient worker who will give up her job and return to honor her role as wife and mother as soon as the war ends.

Nevertheless, in World Wars I and II, most battles did not happen in the United States. This means that men could go to war and act as protectors, and women could stay home and be protected. However, since there was no immediate danger to women in the US, there was a great need for exaggerated depictions of the probable dangers by powerful enemies to help men go to war to protect their women at home. During World War II, for example, the US government sponsored a series of films. In these films, the enemy was depicted as a soldier, either Japanese or German, or a male leader often depicted as Hitler, who would assault, rape, and massacre the women if American soldiers would not fight to protect their women. These depictions of imagined threats to the lives of American women needing protection provided and strengthened the gender system and the unfair distribution of power that has already existed.

Even though American women did not contribute to war efforts at the same level as Europeans during World War I, American women debated and demanded to be accepted as full citizens if they had to work outside their homes. Interestingly, the 19th Amendment allowing American women the right to vote was granted in 1918, before the war ended, and was implemented as law in 1920. Furthermore, even though there was the reinstitution of firm gender roles after World War II, the intensification of women's involvement in paid work caused a change in consciousness that impacted women's progress 20 years later. Some researchers believe that the unexpected abandonment of wartime opportunities for some women was one of the chief promoters of the feminist movement in the 1960s.

One of World War II's most critical gender legacies was consciousness-raising about the importance of the nuclear family and women's prescribed roles as wives and mothers. During the Cold War, the stability of the homeland, state security, and the dominance of the Americans over the Soviets made this phenomenon even stronger. This model symbolized a debate between the

US and Soviet president depicting the American system with homemakers free not to work compared to the Soviet women forced to work outside their home.

The most violent but simultaneously positive era in American history is civil rights movements overlapping with the US participation in the Vietnam War. Inquiries and consciousness about racial justice, class inequalities, gender disparity, and the connotations of manliness were energetically deliberated. Men who could fight in Vietnam but could not vote protested and made it possible to adjust the voting age from 21 to 18. This is a period when many young men participated in thoughtful discussions about what it means to be a man and some of their obligations and rights. Many men started discussing the war as illegitimate during the Vietnam antiwar movement. Thus, there was a conscious and robust connection between male social responsibility, citizenship, manhood, and military service for the first time.

It was also apparent that the Vietnam War legacy was gendered since many did not choose to go to war as the rite of passage to manhood, and those who returned from the war were shamed and not celebrated. In the Persian Gulf war of 1991, however, the United States tried to eliminate the legacy of Vietnam and did win the war. Nonetheless, the Gulf War brought to the forefront some specific new questions about the gendered nature of war and the roles of men and women during times of war in the framework of the gender-unified military.

Theorizing Violence, Power, Peace, Protection, and Justice

There has been a serious effort by feminists globally in challenging us to reconsider phenomena such as violence, power, control, peace, safety, fairness, and integrity to reanalyze the gendered aspects of the experiences of women and men in war zones. This reexamining of the war helps create a context for peace and conflict resolution. Feminist conceptualization of these fundamental issues signifies a critical movement forward about gender during war and the outcome. Some of the central tenets of war are violence, power, protection, peace, and justice. The following section theorizes the relationship between these concepts and gendered war.

Violence. The initial feminist position on violence focused mainly on direct physical violence associated with men and nonviolence associated with women. The feminist perspective became more complicated as they started to analyze the links between violence against women and fundamental culturally sanctioned forms of violence, including the complexity of war and its impact on men's and women's relationships (Sachs *et al.*, 2007; Shalhoub-Kevorkian, 2009; Sharoni *et al.*, 2016). This change in perspective in feminist belief to reanalyze differences helped with a better understanding of the complexity of violence. It became more contextual and relevant to specific struggles tackling systemic abuses of people's rights and respect based on the intersection of gender, race, ethnicity, class, and sexual orientation and not just the casual and linear relationship between gender and war. This characterizations of violence as a multidimensional and intersectional phenomenon has aided researchers and policymakers to have a different outlook about examining violence and its root causes. This includes unfair disparities and unequal power relations fueling violence.

Power. The paradigm of power politics related to international political affairs has been deconstructed and critiqued by feminists for many decades now. They have challenged the notion of power being based on competition, control, domination, and violence, deteriorating into full-blown wars (Sharoni *et al.*, 2016). Michel Foucault's philosophy has influenced feminists to connect with other poststructuralists in treating power as a distinct discourse generating and defining the meaning of everything we do (Shepherd, 2008). Power dynamics impact all aspects of our lives. It is highly gendered, racialized, and saturated with controlled disparities. This intricate and multidimensional conceptualization of power can greatly impact conflicts' evaluation, assessment, and outcome.

Protection. Combining protection and safety with national security that has always been part of the political power has been challenged by feminist researchers and advocates. They have challenged the notion that countries devote tremendous amounts of resources and forces in building a strong military and then, depending on the threat of utilizing the army, protect their people. Many have argued that countries' military power is not providing security and protection, but they become the primary source of insecurity for women and marginalized groups (Scuzzarello, 2008). Therefore, the more governments become obsessed with their military power to protect their national security, the more insecure and unprotected the marginalized communities feel (Abdo & Ronit, 2002; Sachs *et al.*, 2007). Feminists have also discussed that governments utilize the demands for protection to support violent military operations and international expansions. The abundant evidence related to the post-September 11 has made this argument even stronger (Jiwani, 2009; Riley *et al.*, 2008). Feminist reevaluation of this notion of protection demands a shift in belief about security only in terms of national security and challenges us to think about human or global security.

Feminists go beyond analyzing issues related to national security and focus on it as an ever-encompassing patriarchal system that cannot accept a lack of control. They view it as an elusive process with complexities needing to be negotiated and reexamined because historical and sociopolitical circumstances change.

Peace. True peace should not be defined as the absence of just physical violence. It should be defined as the absence of all kinds of violence, such as structural and cultural violence. It should be based on the manifestation of justice and equality (Confortini, 2006), even though peace should be perceived as a definite good that is always more desirable than war. However, some feminists argue that peace should not have a rigid meaning and must be considered a political phenomenon (Shepherd, 2008). The definition of peace should be based on a distinct sociopolitical context and levels of devotion to social and political change. This interpretation challenges us to question whose lives the signing of a peace treaty is prone to enhance and what forms of discrimination and unfairness will be demolished or still be endorsed.

Justice. The serious and continuous feminist attempts to speculate about justice within the context of war and what happens after the war is new in feminist writings (Sharoni *et al.*, 2016). Earlier reports were more focused on advocating for eliminating inequality and implementing social policies to obtain gender justice (Fraser, 2013). The transitional justice frameworks advocating for women's rights as human rights have been part of this discourse. They have asserted that redefining justice should depend on the surviving experiences of women in war zones while being attentive to gender-based harms and evaluating its short- and long-term destructive influences (Bell, 2009; Bell & O'Rourke, 2007).

Feminists have challenged us to redefine concepts like violence, peace, protection, and justice and take the daily efforts of women worldwide into great consideration. Overall, feminist analyses of women's lived experiences in the war zone cannot be restricted to discourse in academia (Giles, 2008) and should be based on the vastly distinct experiences of men and women during war. It should include gender, race, class discrimination, human rights exploitations, assaults on cultural identities, economic development, environmental deprivation, and ecological contexts (Agathangelou & Ling, 2004; Lind, 2010).

The Intersectionality of Gender and War on Women

As has been repeatedly argued in this book, gender identities and relations are socially constructed, and masculine and feminine identities depend on the cultural context and change over time. Third-wave feminists, gays and lesbians, women of color, and working-class women advocates have long been interested in exploring the strong linkage between sexism, racism, colonialism, and homophobias as systems of oppression that strengthen each other based on domination. It is a successful system because it creates a dichotomy between "us" and "them," easily justifying the power and even violence by one group against the "other." Thus, intersectionality is described as the interrelation of gendered selves, dominance, prejudice, oppression, mistreatment, and violence (Davis, 1983; Crenshaw, 1991; Mohanty, 2003). The theories related to intersectionality are based on the experiences of women of color, lesbians, working-class women, arguing that White feminists did not even mention their histories and struggles in Europe and North America. They argued that their experiences were formed by colonialism, race, culture, ethnicity, class, and sexual orientation, along with other aspects of their lived experiences. Women of color in the US asserted that they could not choose between sexism and racism and urged feminists to devote themselves to ending both sexism and racism (hooks, 1984, 1990; Collins, 1991).

Moreover, Southern American women fighting for women's liberation were fighting for national independence and started examining the relationships between gender subjugation and the broader political situation (Mohanty,

1991). This intersectional examination can be very helpful to reveal how the systemic unbalanced distribution of power and privilege can violently spread and increase political issues ending in war. Thus, we must consider third-wave feminist theories of intersectionality to explore the linkage between war and gender and other aspects of women's identities.

The Intersectionality of Gender and War on Men

The impact of men's character and conduct on women, society, and national and international politics has been broadly examined over the years (Zalewski & Parpart, 1998, 2008; Whitworth, 2004). However, crucial research on masculinity, particularly on men's experiences in war and its outcome, is relatively recent. For years the scholarship about men and war signified men's inherent and biological tendency towards violence and, subsequently, war (Hartstock,1989). As a result, men and masculinity were nonetheless habitually and unconsciously considered simple and homogeneous entities.

However, more recent research about men and masculinities takes a fundamental look at the domination of men within international relations (Zalewski, 1998; Zalewski & Parpart, 1998 and 2008). Therefore, the relationship between men, military, and hegemonic masculinity has been examined for wars to be fought across the globe (Whitworth, 2004; Belkin, 2012; Eichler, 2011; Duncanson, 2013; Welland, 2013). The main issue is that masculinities, femininities, and dominant and subordinate masculinities called hegemonic masculinity need to be examined as relational concepts. The relationship between masculinity and femininity and dominant and subordinate masculinities called hegemonic masculinity needs to be examined. This hegemonic masculinity symbolizes one form of cross-culturally elevated masculinity. The main problem with hegemonic masculinity is that it strengthens male power for one group of men but simultaneously subordinates and even culturally denounces other types of masculinities outside of its prohibited borders. In North America, hegemonic masculinity is associated with being White, heterosexual, and socioeconomically and educationally advantaged.

Feminist research about men and masculinities in relation to militarization and war uncovers how qualities and attributes like power, domination, bravery, and violence are encouraged and supported by armed forces and insurgency groups that are dependent on soldiers to fight, as well as communities that approve traditional ideas related to masculinity and femininity during the war (Cockburn & Zarkov, 2002). It seems apparent that the concepts pertaining to military masculinities are critical for turning men into soldiers. This becomes vital to perpetuate violence in international politics, influencing incidents of wartime sexual violence (Baaz & Stern, 2009), torture (Richter-Montpetit, 2007), and constant sexual orientation intolerance and persecution in military settings (Woodward & Winter, 2007).

The Interconnection between Political Violence and Sexual Violence

Feminist research has examined the link between violence against women and a set of complicated sociopolitical and cultural norms contributing to the use of violence. A closer analysis reveals how possession of small arms has influenced intimate-partner violence as well as higher rates of violence against women during and after wars. Feminists have long argued that the warlike explanations of the importance of national security, which leads to the substantial presence of armed forces and police officers, have ironically increased the feelings of uncertainty for women and minority groups (Cockburn & Zarkov, 2002; Sharoni, 2008). Furthermore, militarism, sexual assault, rape, and intimate-partner violence before intensifying a political conflict with another country impact the gender-based violence during the conflict (Sharoni, 2016). Similarly, the pervasiveness of violence against women during the war tends to influence women's life experiences and safety after the war. Even though prior to the 1990s, not much attention was given to rape during war, there is abundant historical evidence that using rape is not simply a recent phenomenon (Buss, 2009). All through history, militarism has facilitated and regulated gender-based crimes committed against women during war. It is essential to add that while sexual assault and rape occur in many societies that are not at war, the pervasiveness and extent of sexual attacks on women significantly increase during the war. These attacks, in some instances, subjugate thousands of women to intentional, premeditated, and systematic rape. In more than 51 countries in Africa, Asia, the Americas, the Middle East, and Europe, sexual violence has been extensively present over the last 20 years (Bastick *et al.*, 2007).

Based on the investigation by the United Nations and by international humanitarian and human rights agencies that have researched the influence of armed conflict on women, the pervasiveness of multiple rapes of women in many war zones has been substantiated (Kirby, 2013). The organized and intentional sexual violence against women was done by different groups of men, involving gangs, local and regional soldiers, organized armed forces, even the United Nations peacekeepers (Whitworth, 2004). The incidents of rape happened in women's own homes, refugee camps, and prisons. In some situations, some women were kept with the militia groups to sexually serve fighting men, while in other cases, sexual slavery became part of the norm (Yoshimi, 2002). Further, the prevalence of sexual assault in the military and the lack of liability of offenders have been the cause of considerable concern in the United States (Hunter, 2007; Nagel, 2014). The use of rape and sexual violence has been a widespread facet of war in history. However, the expression 'rape as a weapon of war' was extensively used by many different groups only during the 1990s, when there was a clear indication about the extensive use of rape and sexual assault in Bosnia (Salzman, 1998).

Later, closer attention to the predominance of gender-based sexualized violence in other war zones such as Liberia, the Democratic Republic of Congo,

Rwanda, and Sierra Leone, became a significant phenomenon (Bastick *et al.*, 2007; Baaz & Stern, 2013; Cohen, 2013). Thus, the categorization of rape and many other forms of gender-based violence is recognized by international policymakers as war crimes. Consequently, in recent years, gender-based violence has become an important concern for the United Nations and many other human rights organizations (Kirby, 2013, 2015). A modest but developing research is now focused on men's experiences during the war, mostly about being exposed to sexualized violence as victims (Nagel & Feitz, 2008).

The Impact of Gender Mainstreaming and War

In 1995, at the Fourth World Conference on Women in Beijing, gender mainstreaming, which focuses on recognizing gender differences impacting global policies and outcomes, was examined (True, 2003). Over the years, various governments, the European Union, the Nordic Council of Ministers, the United Nations, and the Organization for Economic Co-operation and Development also embraced gender mainstreaming as an international policy to achieve gender equality on a much larger global scale (United Nations, 1997; Council of Europe, 1998; True, 2003).

In the year 2000, "Women, Peace, and Security," focusing on international security, was passed unanimously by the United Nations Security Council Resolution 1325. Historically, this is a critical event since it was the first time the United Nations Security Council interconnected women and gender with peace and security (Cohn, 2008). It was also an important development since it suggested including women in decision-making to prevent, manage, and resolve wartime conflicts and advocate for human rights and gender-based violence (Pratt, 2013; United Nations Security Council, 2000).

Furthermore, in the year 2000, the Department of Peacekeeping, in a paper called "Mainstreaming a Gender Perspective in Multidimensional Peace Operations" (United Nations, 2000), clearly echoed 1325's fundamental claim that women's participation in peacekeeping plans improved ceasefire discussions. The UNSCR 1325 has been a major development for women across the globe due to its overt acknowledgment of gendered power relations and women as vital members of the peace process and post-war reconstruction. It highlighted the importance of women's role in peacebuilding and safeguarding women and girls from wartime sexual violence. It also contested the notion that women are only victimized by war and violence and cannot have a sense of agency to change their lives; circumstances for the better (Cohn *et al.*, 2004; Hill *et al.*, 2004). The year after 1325 was passed, several other resolutions were approved to strengthen the aims of the main resolution.

Nevertheless, even though the passing of the resolution has been celebrated by women and men in many parts of the world, the main concern is its execution and long-term influence on related and prospective policies. Other concerns are about transforming the resolution into tangible actions. According to Cohn *et al.* (2004), there seem to be more than a few obstacles to the execution of

1325, including governments not committing to implementing it appropriately, lack of monetary investment and support, and failure to reflect critically to endorse gender mainstreaming (Cohn in Hill *et al.*, 2004). Thus, postcolonial feminists questioned the 1325 resolution as a significant achievement for the global women's movement (Harrington, 2011; Pratt, 2013). According to Pratt (2013), the resolution is not a constructive step toward changing women's and men's lives in war. It depicts yet another engraving of racial and sexual borders related to the political economy of colonialism. Pratt (2013) emphasizes the fact that the passing of the resolution actually helps to continue to formally acknowledge the threat of "dangerous brown men" to keep women and children safe in war zones (p. 779), confirming and legitimizing the need for international interventions and normalizing gendered, raced, and sexualized hierarchies.

In summary, this discourse about the complexity of war and the intersectionality of women's and men's lives should provide a deeper understanding for us always to be attentive to the gender processes at the level of the personal, societal, national, and global for policy building. Research about the impact of war exposes the unbalanced and gendered effects of conflicts. More and more, national governments, international institutions, and organizations are identifying the vital impact of gender on international politics. This discourse should create more space for research and shine a light on the effects of war and violence globally by attending to those who have traditionally been excluded from this debate and ignored and sidelined, including those in Global South, LGBTQT communities, racial and ethnic minorities, and immigrants and refugees.

While we must appreciate the extensive and profound work of many scholars on gender and war, we need to remain aware of many tasks demanding our attention. We need to pay critical attention to policies and advocacy efforts on gender and war for a transnational and critical discourse about gender-sensitive analysis of war. The creation and distribution of innovative knowledge about gender and war will not be meaningful and influential unless we are willing to acknowledge the strains between the Global North and South; between academicians, policymakers, relief workers, advocates; and people whose lives have been destroyed by war and violence, and destructive foreign policies.

The Healing Power of Psychotherapy

Wars have greatly influenced psychiatric history. During the twentieth century and after World Wars, the psychological influences of wars were examined, and the National Institute of Mental Health in the US was established. Most importantly, the variations in soldiers' psychological warning signs created a context for our better awareness of the psychiatric responses to stress. Since the end of World Wars I and II, wars and conflicts have continued to be part of human experience for the last 60 years, with 22 countries in the Eastern region of the world being severely impacted (Murthy & Lakshminarayana, 2006). According to the World Health Organization (WHO), 80 percent of the people in these regions are either currently at war or have experienced war within the last few decades (Ghosh *et al.*, 2004).

War has disastrous and catastrophic consequences for the health and security of people. Research has revealed that wars are linked to more death and disability than any illness. Most importantly, war devastates the livelihood of communities and families and frequently destroys the growth of the collective community and financial structure of countries. War has severe and harmful long-term consequences for children and adults' physical and psychological well-being and social capital. Loss of life in wars is only one of the impacts of conflicts in a region. The real impacts are rampant impoverishment, starvation, disability, financial and collective deterioration, and psychological ailments. Thus, it is impossible to better understand the impact of war on human psychological functioning without considering the multitude of issues that develop because of war. The following section reviews some research that has been done in war-torn countries in Eastern Europe and the Middle East as a very small sample of the impact of the war on children and families.

War and Mental Health

Afghanistan. Instability and destruction have been part of Afghanis' lives since 1978, first with Russia's invasion of their country and then for the last two decades with the United States. This has undoubtedly had painful and pervasive consequences for human anguish and the dislocation of Afghanis devastated by the destruction of their homelands. In a research study examining the mental health of Afghani, investigators found 67.7 percent of participants were dealing with symptoms of depression, 72.2 percent with symptoms of anxiety, and 42 percent with post-traumatic stress disorder. Those that were incapacitated during the war and women had the worse mental health condition (Cardozo *et al.*, 2004). Another study showed that among 1,011 participants above age 15, about 50 percent suffered from traumatic incidents, 39 percent endorsed symptoms of depression, 52 percent anxiety, and 2 percent post-traumatic stress disorder (Scholte *et al.*, 2004). Women exhibited higher rates of mental health symptoms than men. Family and religion were the only sources of support in both studies.

Bosnia. Several studies in this region examining the mental health of people older than 15 revealed the strong association between psychiatric disorders of depression and PTSD and disability. One study stated that 89 percent of men and 90 percent of women conveyed intense feelings of hatred about the Serbs (Mollica *et al.*, 2001). Among 2,796 children who were between 9 and 14 years of age, symptoms of PTSD and grief were very apparent. The findings were associated with the extent and nature of experience, with girls reporting higher distress levels than boys (Smith *et al.*, 2002).

Iraq. The recent history of Iraq is saturated with conflicts. They dealt with several cycles of coups in the 1960s, the war between Iran and Iraq from1980 to 1988, and the anti-Kurdish war between 1986 and1989. In 1991, the Iraqi attack on Kuwait caused the Gulf War, and then in 2003, US and UK forces invaded Iraq, and the war lasted until 2011. The United Nations imposed an economic embargo after the Gulf War, which had an overwhelming influence on the health of Iraqis (Amowitz *et al.*, 2004). A study on 45 Kurdish families residing in refugee camps in Iraq revealed that 87 percent of children and 60 percent of adults had symptoms of PTSD (Ahmad *et al.*, 2000). Another study examining the depressive and trauma symptoms of 84 Iraqi male refugees revealed that a more significant predictor of these mental health symptoms was poor social support (Gorst-Unsworth & Goldenberg, 1998).

Lebanon. The civil war from 1975 to 1990, and the Israeli invasion of Lebanon in 1978 and 1982, have impacted the mental health of many civilians and military personnel. A study conducted in Beirut assessed the link between a mother's distress and children's mental health. They found that the intensity of war-related events is strongly associated with greater degrees of mothers' depressive symptoms. Further, the mother's level of depressive symptoms was the most significant predictor of her child's illness (Bryce *et al.*, 1989). Another research study with 224 Lebanese children ages 10 to 16 revealed that children's traumatic war experiences were positively correlated with PTSD symptoms (Macksoud & Aber, 1996).

Palestine. For a few decades now, a substantial number of research studies from Palestine have informed the field about children and adolescents, women, refugees, and prisoners suffering from increasing psychological damage. Children between the ages of 10 to 19 were part of a study led by the Gaza Community Mental Health Program. The result uncovered that 33 percent of these children endured symptoms of PTSD demanding psychological intervention, 49 percent had moderate PTSD symptoms, 16 percent mild PTSD symptoms, and just less than 2.5 percent had no symptoms. Boys had higher rates at 58 percent compared to girls at 42 percent, and 84 percent of children residing in refugee camps experienced PTSD symptoms compared to 16 percent living in cities (Mousa & Madi, 2003). Another study examined the living conditions of Palestinians and discovered that 46 percent of parents stated showing forceful actions, which negatively impacted their children's academic performance, 27 percent of children had issues with bed-wetting, and 39 percent confirmed that their children agonized by disturbing nightmares. The study also revealed that more than 53 percent of children in refugee camps compared with 41 percent living in cities showed aggressive behaviors. Among these children, 38 percent stated that seeing others being shot was the primary reason influencing their behavior; 34 percent stated watching violence on TV; 7 percent mentioned being restrained at home and not being able to go out; and 11 percent stated the impact of detention and beating of family members, loved ones and neighbors impacted their aggressive behavior. More than 70 percent of the participants informed researchers that they did not receive any psychological assistance for the difficulties their children were experiencing (Sarraj & Qouta, 2005). It seemed that the most widespread forms of trauma children experienced were related to witnessing funerals for 95 percent of these children, witnessing shooting for 83 percent, watching injured or dead strangers for 67 percent, and witnessing family members being injured or killed for 62 percent. Girls showed more vulnerability and psychological symptoms (Mousa & Madi, 2003).

Based on the review of these studies, it is possible to conclude that women have a heightened level of susceptibility to the psychological outcomes of war, and distress levels directly impact their children's mental health. Further, mothers' level of depression during the pre- and post-natal periods can be a strong predictor for poorer infants' growth. There is also a strong association between social support underpinning maternal psychosocial health and a linkage between gender-based violence and mental disorders in war-stricken territories. There has also been a recognition of women's resiliency despite their vulnerability and stress, which has impacted their role in supporting their families. The research has also consistently shown that there are much higher rates of psychological problems in children directly related to war-related trauma they have experienced. The important research done in Palestine reveals that adolescents are the most susceptible to psychological disorders out of all different age groups. Researchers consistently emphasize the importance of mental health services, social support, religion, and cultural practices to lower the risks of war-related traumas.

Individual Impact of War

Humans do not respond the same way to stressful events, even though somatic symptoms are subjective experiences produced by war and its disturbances globally. People often have enough psychological awareness to know that their symptoms are stress-related. Still, somatic symptoms are so prevalent in war-torn regions because it is the conventional mode for seeking help from the medical system without the stigma attached to their mental health issues. Some researchers perceive somatic warning signs as physical responses propelled by stress. In contrast, others emphasize their communicational component, which might be the only accessible manifestations of the communal distress of defenseless and oppressed people deprived of social and economic compensation. While the effect of war on soldiers has been explored, the medical information on noncombatants has proliferated only in the past few decades.

Nevertheless, it is built primarily on clinical populations of refugees who live in the Western hemisphere. Over the past 30 years, research studies have been centered around understanding and helping those with systems of posttraumatic stress disorder. Even though PTSD seems to be a common disorder internationally when people are impacted by war, the notion that this Western-based diagnostic category depicts the fundamental nature of human reaction to traumatic events in any circumstance and any context, irrespective of particular social and cultural context, is debatable. Characteristics of posttraumatic stress disorder are often the byproduct of what is happening to survivors. It is not what survivors consider important since they continue to function despite facing endless adversity and danger. Consequently, the naïve utilization of diagnostic specifications for post-traumatic stress disorder may substantially increase the number of people needing therapy and treatment.

It is apparent that some victims develop considerable psychiatric and relational dysfunction. Still, there is not a clear correlation between traumatic incidents and after-effects, as perhaps a prewar history of psychological vulnerability can be a risk factor (Tanielian & Jaycox, 2008). Research indicates that the impact of war on family, society, and financial aspects of life can be very significant predictors of psychological symptoms (Basoglu *et al.*, 1994). In a study examining the depressive symptoms of Iraqi asylum seekers in England, inadequate social support had a more significant impact on their depression than a history of torture (Gorst & Goldenberg, 1998). Indisputably, the existence of a stable and supportive community is a significant protective factor and can be a source of support. The apparent impact of family attachment and other sources of support in safeguarding the effects of war on children can also be essential.

Further, research reveals that children's psychological health remains relatively stable if adult caregivers can manage adversities in their situation. Bodily injury or disability has also been perceived as a risk factor for developing emotional symptoms but cannot be listed as the sole factor. Other relational factors may be more relevant for developing these disorders beyond individual reactions to trauma.

Collective Impact of War

The common perception of trauma is in accordance with the conventional practice of psychology in which individuals are the unit of analysis, and healing is a personal experience. However, war is not a secluded encounter, and the anguish it produces impacts everyone and can only be solved in a social context. The most critical way to deal with horrendous war experiences is to understand their social significance and meaning in terms of mystical, religious, and political reasons. Thus, victims of war must often deal with incomprehensible events that make them feel helpless and unsure about everything they used to believe about human kindness. The worst aspect of war is how it affects the entire collective structure of a society and can destroy people's support and adaptation. Fear produces suspicion and, as expected, diminishes a sense of community, which can have other negative consequences. There are times they have to witness the destruction of their history and cultural identity.

On the other hand, people subjected to political aggression are not always simply victims who cannot react to their situation. Even children may not be passive onlookers without a good understanding of the causes of their victimization. Therefore, psychotherapists must go beyond an individually based impact of war and view the war from a systemic and collective perspective.

Mental Health Interventions

Cultural norms, belief systems, and customs create a context for governmental health standards globally. However, Western psychological norms and practices have been part of the worldwide expansion of Western philosophy claiming that it is the ultimate knowledge and much more sophisticated than the local knowledge and expertise of people impacted by war. In many of these war-torn regions, the biopsychological model based on the Western clinical psychiatric models may not be helpful. Experts consulting with the World Health Organization and UNICEF have stated that the outbreaks of posttraumatic stress disorder and the early intervention using the Western mental health model is at best a very short-term healing solution. It does not prevent the later onset of other mental health disorders or new cycles of violence in vulnerable war zones (Summerfield, 1999). There is not much research done to review the efficacy of these interventions.

Most importantly, the typical reaction to a disastrous situation perceived as a mental health disorder views people as passive victims instead of active survivors. It tends to ignore the strength and resiliency of these groups. These borrowed Western models of mental health often do not recognize the impact of social actions and empowerment in promoting psychological health. The main push for these caring interventions should be toward the war debilitated societal structure for those who survive the atrocities and promote psychological resilience and regaining strengths for all. Survivors must be helped to reclaim their pride and have a better sense of control over their situation. They need to rebuild their connections to their society's cultural, social, and economic foundations the way it makes sense to them. Eventually, people recover from atrocities of war not because they received help as mentally ill but as active, dignified, and empowered people. Psychotherapists should advocate for refugees with pro-family interventions, including employment opportunities and community-based help for children to regain a more positive sense of self. Children may often act out or play out war-related themes to make sense of events that happened around them. This should not be viewed as symptoms of posttraumatic stress disorder, even though frequent interaction with teachers and health care workers could support the acknowledgment and management of those needing mental health services.

Refuges who relocate to Western countries may need even more mental health services since few support systems are available. Some refugees receive unsuitable and irrelevant psychiatric diagnoses due to the host culture's lack of understanding of important cross-cultural issues. Additionally, these unique challenges interrupt their normal life courses, there is loss of social and financial status, the hostility of the host culture, and isolation in a strange culture for which there are no therapeutic remedies. While psychotropic medication may be a short-term solution, survivors of traumatic events do much better if they have appropriate and supportive psychotherapy.

Moreover, when it comes to the aftermath of war, history has shown that social restructuring, public acknowledgment, and restoration of justice, if possible are much better medicine to help victims of war recover from violence they have experienced. In war, health and sickness have social and political origins. Posttraumatic reactions are not just a personal reaction to a painful situation needing personal recovery and adjustment. It is the prosecution of the sociopolitical powers that created them. Refugees often need health care professionals to reveal their political standing before trusting them. The psychotherapist must be able to go beyond their traditional neutral stands and be ready not to be morally and politically impartial. They also need to be able to acknowledge clients' broader rights. All military and powerful financial leaders protect ingrained social inequalities in their countries with weapons bought from the West under the disguise of national defense.

In a study by Sivard, in 1989, the mean spending per capita on weapons in developing countries was $38 instead of $12 on health. This trend has become even more significant over the year. The sad news is that all the world's leading exporters of weapons are major players on the United Nations Security Council. Thus, the Western-led global hierarchy based on military power and the need for extensive financial gains significantly offset concerns related to human rights and justice for masses of the least protected individuals on the planet. Western psychotherapists can support refugees' mental health needs by at least acknowledging the pain and suffering as well as the resilience of those seeking psychological help. As psychotherapists, we must separate our loyalties to a political system that is the source of oppression for many developing nations, from loyalties to those we serve.

Conclusion

Over the years, all around the world, theorizing about war and peace and the psychological impact of war has become more complicated. Combining the term gender with women and encapsulating gender differences by considering men as combatants and women as peacemakers have not offered a useful understanding of between-group differences. The postmodern theories have moved beyond basically assessing and making distinctions between the experiences of men and women in war. We must understand that gender is fundamental to character development and change across cultures and contexts and greatly influences our perception of war and its consequences. We should no longer emphasize the fact that gender matters. We should concentrate on how gender influences war's political beliefs and practices.

References

Abdo, N. A., & Ronit, L. (2002). *Women and the Politics of Military Confrontation.* Indiana University Press.

Agathangelou, A. M., & Ling, H. M. (2004). Power, borders, security, wealth: Lessons of violence and desire from September 11. *International Studies Quarterly, 48*(3),517–538.

Ahmad, A., Sofi, M. A., Sundelin-Wahlsten, V., & Von Knorring, A. L. (2000). Post-traumatic stress disorder in children after the military operation "Anfal" in Iraqi Kurdistan. *European Child & Adolescent Psychiatry, 9*(4), 235–243.

Amowitz, L. L., Kim, G., Reis, C., Asher, J. L., & Iacopino, V. (2004). Human rights abuses and concerns about women's health and human rights in southern Iraq. *Jama, 291*(12), 1471–1479.

Baaz, M. E., & Stern, M. (2009). Why do soldiers rape? Masculinity, violence and sexuality in the armed forces in the Congo (DRC). *International Studies Quarterly, 53*(2), 495–518.

Baaz, M. E., & Stern, M. (2013). *Sexual Violence as a Weapon of War?: Perceptions, prescriptions, problems in the Congo and Beyond.* New York: Zed Books.

Basoglu, M., Paker, M., Ozmen, E., Tasdemir, O., & Sahin, D. (1994). Factors related to long-term traumatic stress in survivors of torture in Turkey. *Jama, 272*(5), 357–363.

Bastick, M., Grimm, K., & Kunz, R. (2007). *Sexual Violence in Armed Conflict: Global Overview and Implications for the Security Sector.* Geneva: Centre for the Democratic Control of Armed Forces.

Belkin, A. (2012). *Bring Me Men: Military Masculinity and the Benign Façade of American Empire 1898–2001.* London: Hurst.

Bell, C. (2009). Transitional justice, interdisciplinarity, and the state of the 'field' or 'non-field.' *International Journal of Transitional Justice, 3*(1): 5–27.

Bell, C., & O'Rourke, C. (2007). Does feminism need a theory of transitional justice? An introductory essay. *International Journal of Transitional Justice, 1*(1): 23–44.

Bryce, J. W., Walker, N., Ghorayeb, F., & Kanj, M. (1989). Life experiences, response styles and mental health among mothers and children in Beirut, Lebanon. *Social Science and Medicine, 28*(7), 685–695.

Buss, D. E. (2009). Rethinking "rape as a weapon of war." *Feminist Legal Studies, 17*(2), 145–163.

Cardozo, B. L., Bilukha, O. O., Crawford, C. A. G., Shaikh, I., Wolfe, M. I., Gerber, M. L., & Anderson, M. (2004). Mental health, social functioning, and disability in postwar Afghanistan. *Jama, 292*(5): 575–584.

Cockburn, C., & Zarkov, D. (Eds). (2002). *The Postwar Moment: Militaries, Masculinities and International Peacekeeping.* London: Lawrence and Wishart.

Cohen, D. K. (2013). Explaining rape during civil war: Cross-national evidence (1980–2009). *American Political Science Review, 107*(3), 461–477.

Cohn, C. (2008). Mainstreaming gender in UN security policy: a path to political transformation?. In S. Rai & G. Waylen (Eds.), *In Global Governance: Feminist Perspectives.* Basingstoke: Palgrave Macmillan.

Cohn, C., Kinsella, H., & Gibbings, S. (2004). Women, peace and security, Resolution 1325. *International Feminist Journal of Politics, 6*(1), 130–140.

Collins, P. H. (1991). *Black Feminist Thought: Knowledge, Consciousness, and the Politics of Empowerment.* London: Routledge.

Confortini, C. (2006). Galtung, violence, and gender: the case for a peace studies/feminism alliance. *Peace and Change, 31*(3): 333–367.

Council of Europe. (1998). *Gender Mainstreaming: Conceptual Framework, Methodology and Presentation of Good Practices*. Final report of activities of the group of specialists on mainstreaming (Rapporteur Group on the Equality Between Women and Men, GR-EG). Committee of Ministers.

Crenshaw, K. (1991). Mapping the margins: intersectionality, identity politics, and violence against women of color. *Stanford Law Review*, *43*, 1241–1299.

Davis, A. (1983). *Women, Race and Class*. New York: Random House.

Dull, J. R. (1985). *A Diplomatic History of the American Revolution*. New Haven, CT: Yale University Press.

Duncanson, C. (2013). *Forces for Good? Military Masculinities and Peacebuilding in Afghanistan and Iraq*. Basingstoke: Palgrave Macmillan.

Eichler, M. (2011). *Militarizing Men: Gender, Conscription, and War in Post-Soviet Russia*. Stanford, CA: Stanford University Press.

El-Sarraj, E., & Qouta, S. (2005). The Palestinian experience. In López-Ibor, J. J., Christodoulou, G., Maj, M., Sartorius, N. & Okasha, A. (Eds), *Disasters and Mental h Health* (pp. 229–238). Chichester: Wiley.

Encyclopedia.com. (2018). https://www.encyclopedia.com/social-sciences-and-law/political-science-and-government/military-affairs-nonnaval/war#1O126War

Fraser, N. (2013). Reframing justice in a globalizing world. In *Fortunes of Feminism: From State-managed Capitalism to Neoliberal Crisis* (pp. 189–209). London: Verso Books.

Ghosh, N., Mohit, A., & Murthy, R. S. (2004). Mental health promotion in post-conflict countries. *The Journal of the Royal Society for thePromotion of Health*, *124*(6), 268–270.

Giles, W. (2008). Reflections on the women in conflict zones network: lessons from the past and forward-looking possibilities. *International Feminist Journal of Politics*, *10*(1), 102–112.

Gleditsch, N. P., & Hegre, H. (1997). Peace and democracy: Three levels of analysis. *Journal of Conflict Resolution*, *41*(2), 283–310.

Gluck, S. (1987). *Rosie the Riveter Revisited: Women, the War and Social Change*. Boston, MA: Twayne.

Goldstein, J. S. (2001). *War and Gender: How Gender Shapes the War System and vice versa*. Cambridge, UK: Cambridge University Press.

Gorst-Unsworth, C., & Goldenberg, E. (1998). Psychological sequelae of torture and organized violence suffered by refugees from Iraq. Trauma-related factors compared to social factors in exile. *The British Journal of Psychiatry*, *172*(1), 90–94.

Harrington, C. (2011). Resolution 1325 and post-cold war feminist politics. *International Feminist Journal of Politics*, *13*(4), 557–575.

Hartstock, N. (1989). Masculinity, heroism and the making of war. In A. Harris & Y. King (Eds), *Rocking the Ship of the State: Towards a Feminist Peace Politics*. Boulder, CO: Westview.

Hill, F., Cohn, C., and Enloe, C. (2004). UN Security Council Resolution 1325 three years on: gender, security and organizational change. *Center for Gender in Organizations*, 941–80.

hooks, b. (1984). *Feminist Theory: From Margin to Center*. London: Pluto Press.

hooks, b. (1990). *Yearning: Race, Gender and Cultural Politics*. London: Turnaround.

Hunter, M. (2007). *Honor Betrayed: Sexual Abuse in America's Military*. New York: Barricade Books.

Jiwani, Y. (2009). Helpless maidens and chivalrous knights: Afghan women in the Canadian press. *University of Toronto Quarterly*, *78*(2), 728–744.

Kirby, P. (2013). How is rape a weapon of war? Feminist international relations, modes of critical explanation and the study of wartime sexual violence. *European Journal of International Relations, 19*(4), 797–821.

Kirby, P. (2015). Acting time; or, the abolitionist and the feminist. *International Feminist Journal of Politics, 1*(3), 508–513.

Lind, A. (2010). *Development, Sexual Rights and Global Governance*. Abingdon: Routledge.

Macksoud, M. S., & Aber, J. L. (1996). The war experiences and psychosocial development of children in Lebanon. *Child Development, 67*(1), 70–88.

Ministry of Defence. (2020). *UK Armed Forces Biannual Diversity Statistics*. Retrieved from https://assets.publishing.service.gov.uk/government/uploads/system/uploads/attachment_data/file/943009/Biannual_Diversity_Statistics_Publication_Oct20.pdf

Mohanty, C. T. (1991). Cartographies of struggle: third world women and the politics of feminism. In C. T. Mohanty *et al.* (Eds), *Third World Women and the Politics of Feminism*. Indiana University Press.

Mohanty, C. T. (2003). *Feminism Without Borders: Decolonizing Theory, Practicing Solidarity*. Durham, NC: Duke University Press.

Mollica, R. F., Sarajlic, N., Chernoff, M., Lavelle, J., Vuković, I. S., & Massagli, M. P. (2001). Longitudinal study of psychiatric symptoms, disability, mortality, and emigration among Bosnian refugees. *Jama, 286*(5), 546–554.

Moore, E. (2020). *Women in Combat: Five-year status update*. Retrieved from: https://www.cnas.org/publications/commentary/women-in-combat-five-year-status-update

Mousa, F., & Madi, H. (2003). Impact of the humanitarian crisis in the occupied Palestinian territory on people and services. *Gaza: United Nations Relief and Works Agency for Palestinian Refugees in the Near East (UNRWA)*.

Murthy, R. S., & Lakshminarayana, R. (2006). Mental health consequences of war: a brief review of research findings. *World Psychiatry, 5*(1), 25.

Nagel, J. (2014). Rape and war: fighting men and comfort women. In M. Stombler, D. Baunach, W. Simonds, E. Windsor, & E. Burgess (Eds), *Sex Matters: The Sexuality and Society Reader* (pp. 641–648). New York: W.W. Norton.

Nagel, J., & Feitz, L. (2008). The militarization of gender and sexuality in the Iraq war. In H. Carreiras & G. Kümmel (Eds), *Women in the Military and in Armed Conflict* (pp. 201–225). V.S. Verlag für Sozialwissenschaften.

Pratt, N. (2013). Reconceptualizing gender, reinscribing racial-sexual boundaries in international security: the case of UN Security Council Resolution 1325 on "Women, Peace and Security." *International Studies Quarterly, 57*(4), 772–783.

Richter-Montpetit, M. (2007). Empire, desire and violence: a queer transnational feminist reading of the prisoner "abuse" in Abu Ghraib and the question of "gender equality." *International Feminist Journal of Politics, 9*(1), 58–59.

Riley, R., Mohanty, C. T., & Pratt, M. B. (Eds). (2008). *Feminism and War: Confronting US Imperialism*. London: Zed Books.

Sachs, D., Sa'ar, A., & Aharoni, S. (2007). How can I feel for others when I myself am beaten? The impact of the armed conflict on women in Israel. *Sex Roles, 57*(7–8), 593–606.

Salzman, T. A. (1998). Rape camps as a means of ethnic cleansing: religious, cultural, and ethical responses to rape victims in the former Yugoslavia. *Human Rights Quarterly, 20*(2), 348–378.

Scholte, W. F., Olff, M., Ventevogel, P., de Vries, G. J., Jansveld, E., Cardozo, B. L., & Crawford, C. A. G. (2004). Mental health symptoms following war and repression in Eastern Afghanistan. *Jama 292*(5), 585–593..

Scuzzarello, S. (2008). National security versus moral responsibility: An analysis of integration programs in Malmo, Sweden. *Social Politics: International Studies in Gender, State and Society, 15*(1), 5–31.

Shalhoub-Kevorkian, N. (2009). *Militarization and Violence against Women in Conflict Zones in the Middle East: A Palestinian Case-Study*. Cambridge, UK: Cambridge University Press.

Sharoni, S. (2008). De-militarizing masculinities in the age of empire. *The Austrian Political Science Journal (special issue: 'Counter/Terror/Wars: Feminist Perspectives'), 37*(2), 147–164.

Sharoni, S. (2016). Militarism and gender-based violence. In N. Naples, M. Wickramasinghe, & A. W. W. Ching (Eds.), *The Wiley-Blackwell Encyclopedia of Gender and Sexuality Studies* (pp. 1–9). Oxford: Wiley Blackwell.

Sharoni, S., Welland, J., Steiner, L., & Pedersen, J. (2016). *Handbook on Gender and War*. Cheltenham, UK: Edward Elgar.

Shepherd, L. J. (2008). *Gender, Violence and Security: Discourse as Practice*. London: Zed Books.

Sivard, R. L. (1989). *World Military and Social Expenditures*. Washington, DC: World Priorities.

Smith, P., Perrin, S., Yule, W., Hacam, B., & Stuvland, R. (2002). War exposure and children from Bosnia-Herzegovina: Psychological adjustment in a community sample. *Journal Trauma Stress, 15*, 147–156. doi: 10.1023/A:1014812209051. PMID: 12013066.

Summerfield, D. (1999). A critique of seven assumptions behind psychological trauma programmes in waraffected areas. *Social Science & Medicine, 48*, 144–962.

Tanielian, T. L., & Jaycox, L. (2008). *Invisible Wounds of War: Psychological and Cognitive Injuries, Their Consequences, and Services to Assist Recovery* (Vol. I). Santa Monica, CA: Rand Corporation.

True, J. (2003). Mainstreaming gender in global public policy. *International Feminist Journal of Politics, 5*(3), 368–396.

United Nations. (1997). *Report of the Economic and Social Council for 1997*. Report of the Economic and Social Council for 1997.

United Nations. (2000). *Mainstreaming a Gender Perspective in Multidimensional Peace Operations*. Lessons Learned Unit: Department of Peacekeeping Operations, July.

United Nations Security Council. (2000). *Resolution 1325*. Security Council, 31 October.

Welland, J. (2013). Militarised violences, basic training, and the myths of asexuality and discipline. *Review of International Studies, 39*(4), 881–902.

Whitworth, S. (2004). *Men, Militarism & UN Peacekeeping: A Gendered Analysis*. Boulder, CO: Lynne Rienner.

Woodward, R., & Winter, T. (2007). *Sexing the Soldier: The Politics of Gender in the Contemporary British Army*. Abingdon: Routledge.

Yoshimi, Y. (2002). *Comfort Women: Sexual Slavery in the Japanese Military During World War II*. Columbia University Press.

Zalewski, M. (1998). Introduction: from the "woman" question to the "man" question in international relations. In M. Zalewski & J. Parpart (Eds), *The 'Man' Question in International Relations* (pp. 2–13). Boulder, CO: Westview.

Zalewski, M., & Parpart, J. (Eds.). (1998). *The 'Man' Question in International Relations*. Boulder, CO: Westview.

Zalewski, M., & Parpart, J. (Eds) (2008). *Rethinking the Man Question: Sex, Gender and Violence in International Relations*. London: Zed Books.

9 Gender and Violence

Introduction

Violence Against Women (VAW) is a term used to define violence based on prescriptive gender roles that, along with the unequal power relationships between the two genders, happen in a cultural context of a society. Violence impacts women's sense of emotional and physical well-being and their positive contributions to their home life, communities where they reside, and their workplace. Globally about one in five women suffer from the consequences of physical and sexual violence in their intimate relationship or sexual violence from a stranger in their lifetime (World Health Organization, 2021).

Gender-Based Violence (GBV) and Violence Against Women (VAW) have been used interchangeably. However, Violence Against Women is a subcategory of Gender-Based Violence. Gender-Based violence is "Any act of gender-based violence that results in, or is likely to result in, physical, sexual or psychological harm or suffering to women, including threats of such acts, coercion or arbitrary deprivations of liberty, whether occurring in public or private life" (UN Declaration on the Elimination of Violence against Women, 1993).

It is important to say that not all types of violence revolve around gendered power relations, even though all forms of violence are gendered. Many discourses have reassessed the idea that females are always the victims and males are always the villains. There are times and circumstances when women have been the perpetrators. However, based on the research that has been conducted cross-culturally, women and girls fully represent the substantial group of gender-based violence victims, and men represent the majority of perpetrators.

Different Types of Gender-Based Violence

It is sadly apparent that gender-based violence occurs in all cultures and at all phases of women's life-cycle. Baby girls get aborted because having a baby boy is preferred, and women are more likely to be abused at old age. Sexual and physical violence is also prevalent in all cultures, even though some countries

DOI: 10.4324/9781003088189-10

have better laws to protect women. In contrast, other countries do not have any set policies to prevent many types of violence against women. In many societies, women might go through gender-based violence based on who controls their income, social position, profession; cultural background; religious beliefs; and sexual orientation. In a research study with over 24,000 women that lived in 15 cities in 10 countries by the World Health Organization, between 15 to 71 percent of women said they had experienced intimate partner violence (2005). There are other types of violence, such as rape and sexual assault, being used as a weapon of war after significant disasters and when there is an unbalanced ratio of men to women (Reuters Foundation, 2005; Mehta, 2004). Due to these variations in kind, complexities in defining it, and lack of reporting by women, there is not much research to measure the impact of gender-based violence and utilize the findings to promote preventative measures.

The inherent power imbalances between men and women individually and collectively can be one of the primary sources of gender-based violence. Some men routinely use violence to coerce or confine women to provide services for them at the personal, family, community, and societal levels. This can potentially be a human-rights violation or public-health issue stopping women from accessing their economic rights, social responsibilities, cultural contributions, civil duties, and political power. Thus, gender-based violence has been categorized as a fundamental public health issue by the World Health Organization since it has been a direct reason for physical harm, illness, and even death. These types of violence influence women's well-being through unwanted pregnancies and their significant health issues, mental health challenges, sexually transmitted diseases, human immunodeficiency virus (HIV), and acquired Immune Deficiency Syndrome (AIDS). The sexual and intimate violence in Africa due to women and girls' economic, social, and cultural disparities was one of the significant contributors to the HIV and AIDS epidemic (Human Rights Watch, 2002).

Gender-based violence prevents many women from enjoying a long and heartful life and experiencing liberty, respectability, and dignity. When poverty and gender-based violence impact women's lives, it limits women's choices even more. At the family level, it reduces their productivity and impacts their negotiating efforts with their spouses, intensifying their helplessness. It affects their ability to work and be productive at the societal level due to an unsafe work environment. Gender-based violence restricts women's options for impacting positive societal changes. It is a measure of blocked progress for society since it affects women's developmental opportunities in an oppressive and unfair cultural, social, and political environment (United Nations Economic and Social Council Commission on Human Rights (2003)). According to Sen (1999): "there is nothing more important in the political economy of development than the adequate recognition of women's participation and political, economic, and social leadership" (p. 103).

International Progress for Women's Rights

Implementing the Declaration on the Elimination of Violence against Women (1993) is a hopeful step toward preventing violence against women at home, in the community, and at large. The Declaration demands that state officials have contractual obligations to stop, examine, and penalize any violent actions against women. Many non-governmental organizations worldwide, such as the Beijing Platform for Action (2022) and United Nation Security Council Resolution 1325 (2000), fought for years to make violence against women a public human rights issue. The formation of the International Criminal Court (ICC) in 2003 identified extreme violence like rape in armed conflict as a weapon of war and a gender-based crime for the first time. Even though these declarations might appear inaccessible for ordinary women's everyday unpleasant life experiences, these are all significant accomplishments and the absolute first step to reach a higher level of gender justice. Nevertheless, it has been about two decades since the Declaration on the Elimination of Violence against Women has been accepted, and enormous problems still persist for its reliable and successful execution and implementation.

Many countries have already defaulted on their promises under the Beijing Platform for actions to support women's rights, including gender-based violence, due to the lack of a comprehensive political process and a significant restructuring of public resources. Thus, since the international and governmental official plans have been highly inadequate to protect women against different types of violence, many civil-society groups advocating for women's rights are working on these initiatives. The kinds of programs focus on offering protective services to women and girls who suffer from GBV and can also help in reducing future risks. These protective services incorporate utilizing shelters, psychotherapy, and legal services. Prevention tactics consist of challenging governments to create appropriate regulations or reinforce existing legislation to protect women. It should also involve enhancing people's knowledge, mindset, and perception about the impact of gender-based violence using media and public education. Many non-governmental organizations advocating for women's rights employ a comprehensive and ecological analysis of women's context to help them recognize their economic rights to decrease their helplessness in relational conflicts. The most important movement is by non-governmental organizations run by men striving to stop gender-based violence, especially intimate partner and sexual violence. Their approach is helping men understand the impact of gender-based violence, challenging men to question their own thoughts and actions regarding their sense of power and control over women.

The Eradication of Gender-Based Violence

Eliminating violence against women has become a crucial cross-cultural challenge. Women's organizations, international NGOs, and human-rights advocates have successfully named GBV a human-rights abuse and an obstruction to societal progress. Still, there are many obstacles to its implementation.

The heartbreaking truth is that they have barely even scratched the surface in many countries, let alone been destroyed. The main argument still remains that gender-based violence can only be eradicated when extreme gender disparities are significantly decreased, and women can fully obtain different kinds of rights. This can only happen when women have much higher representation in the governments and act as legislators impacting policies and distributions of resources to reduce the vulnerability to gender-based violence.

The so-called "war on terror," after September 11, led by the US and UK governments, triggered local reactions in the Middle East, creating many challenges to women's human rights issues and increasing gender-based violence in many ways. In some countries like Pakistan, India, and Sri Lanka, religious fundamentalists prevent or even oppose women's rights issues (United Nations, 2006). Then there are other religious fundamentalists, particularly the US Christian right, impacting the US government's reproductive health policies in the global South. Therefore, women's rights are jeopardized when a woman is killed in Gaza by the Hamas group, when the Vatican opposed the use of condoms in Africa, or when the Christian rights deny funding to reproductive health organizations in the global South.

Use of technology. The utilization of reproductive technology and information and communications technologies (ICTs) can potentially positively impact women's rights. For example, ultrasound can help women be safer during pregnancy. However, it is also used for sex-selective abortions. Due to the economic advantages of having a son who can provide for parents at old age, sex-selective abortions and female infanticide have been more utilized in South and East Asia, North Africa, and the Middle East. Information and Communication Technology can also have paradoxical functions. GBV offenders can use cyberspace pornography, including child pornography, chat rooms used to abuse children, and video games glorifying violence against women. On the other hand, women's advocacy groups can lobby for policies and coordinate campaigns.

Climate change. Developing countries are excessively impacted by climate change because of severe weather patterns such as hurricanes and floods and long-term changes like famines and increased land saltiness. It is critical to acknowledge that climate change, the task of ecological growth, and poverty-stricken women's human rights, which include freedom from violence, are all strongly tied collectively. Women's unique susceptibility is related to the gendered division of labor, and the type of work women and girls are responsible for doing. For example, if there is a problem accessing clean water, women and girls have to spend many more hours collecting water. When there are water scarcities, there are more water-borne illnesses, and since it is typically women that have to take care of an ill family member, it increases the amount of work they have to do. If impoverished women have to devote most of their time to these types of work, they consequently have less time and energy to work independently to earn an income, learn to read and write or have knowledge about the impact of local politics on their daily lives. Combining these issues influences their rights as humans and enhances their susceptibility to gender-based violence.

Therefore, all projects related to adjusting and alleviating climate change in areas impacting impoverished populations should also strongly support gender equality. There are undoubtedly possibilities for collaboration between different resources. For example, Chynoweth & Patrick (2007) discussed the danger of sexual violence against women when collecting firwoods for cooking in refugee camps. They provided solar cookers to women in these camps to keep them safe from gender-based violence and firewood collection, and to alleviate carbon emissions.

International Strategies

According to the last United Nations report in 2006, out of 192 UN state members, 102 countries do not have a specific official provision on domestic violence. Rape within the context of marriage is not a crime in 53 countries, and only 93 countries have some governmental and judicial requirements against human trafficking. Governments should bring their own laws on gender-based violence into line with their international commitments at the national level.

Moreover, any enhancement in legislation about gender-based violence has to align with corresponding procedures in the criminal justice, health care, and education systems. This change should include coaching judges and police officers, educating healthcare providers, and promoting consciousness-raising curricula using the existing education system.

It has been known that public education campaigns can be the best strategy for reinforcing passing new laws and improving the accountability of the criminal justice system because it creates widespread pressure on governments to respond. In South Asia, for example, Oxfam International advocated against gender-based violence by stating that we need to eliminate the shame and stigma about women dealing with violence. We need to drastically change our assumption that gender-based violence is a private issue. We need to work on recognizing its pervasiveness, working hard to make it intolerable; promote equality in all aspects of men's and women's relationship with each other (Mehta, 2004).

Further, there are severe human rights violations based on sexual orientation, even by governments, sanctioned against lesbians, gay men, bisexuals, and transgenders that go beyond just a binary and one-directional occurrence of violence. According to Leach and Humphreys (2007), there is a great need for systemic studies looking into gender-based violence between men and women, separate from examining violence between men and women. There is also a great need for impact assessment specific to gender-based violence (Kirk, 2007). For example, this kind of research may often involve physical risk for the researcher and women participants. Nevertheless, impact assessment is important because it is correlated with financial support. The private-sector mentality has influenced the way donors support a project needing to see hard evidence in short-term program effectiveness. However, dealing with gender-based violence requires a serious transformation in mindsets and actions, which takes years to work on and is difficult to assess (Hayes, 2007).

Men and Gender-Based Violence

It might seem like an impractical project or a simple-minded plan to think about working with men to prevent gender-based violence since there are very few men eager to take part in prevention projects. However, long-lasting change only happens when men are part of the process since men are the primary perpetrators of violence against women. This sad truth should help us wonder why men often act as aggressors and what can be done to change and eradicate this pattern? Any project working on ending violence against women should examine the cultural factors perpetuating the cycle of violence. The main point should be that men and women together can stop this cycle. This should include engaging men of all ages and educating them about the long-lasting causes of gender-based violence. These programs should engage men in reflecting on the cultural formation of masculine identity and the interactional patterns between men and women. The two primary components impacting gender-based violence are manifestations of masculinity and hierarchical gender relationships. The main issue in violence against women and violent behavior in men is highly connected. Men need to understand that being a man is a risk factor in a gendered relationship, and their emotional understanding of this fact will tremendously help with a paradigm shift.

However, no man can accept that being a man is an inherent risk factor in a relationship if we don't examine all the factors contributing to these risky behaviors. There is no violent gene responsible for men's behavior. They are not innately violent. Masculinity and its behaviors create an environment where acting violently is related to contextual factors and culturally sanctioned patterns of behavior based on images and stereotypes present in men's lives. Nevertheless, knowing that violence is a learned behavior creates hope because the hegemonic cultural ideal of masculinity that causes violence against women is profoundly embedded in our cultural contexts but can be changed since masculine ideals have changed over time and do not impact men the same way.

The socialization process is not the same for all men in all societies, and many men do not use violence against women. They do not think it is an acceptable form of exerting power. In fact, cross-culturally, men themselves have grown up witnessing and experiencing high levels of violence and aggression, and many have been victims themselves. Some may imitate the same familiar violent actions in their own intimate and family relationships. Others may refuse to be part of the same vicious cycle and consider other ways of relating and changing their behaviors, leading to violence. Men who have experienced being a victim of violence can become powerful allies to change societal patterns and help with changing violent behaviors. Governments can pass laws, try to regulate men's behavior, and come up with longer prison sentences for perpetrators. Still, unless men develop the proper skills to use nonviolent channels to express their emotions, there is unlikely to be a substantial decline in gender-based violence. Teaching men new skills and changing their perceptions about the use of violence takes time and can be a very gradual process. However, research has shown that once men have more knowledge, they can support the prevention of violence instead of justifying or repeating it.

The prevention of gender violence should include particular attention to men developing critical thinking to promote a healthy discourse, ensuring that their tasks considering preventing violence are emphasized as essential for change. Men that have experienced violence or have been socialized around violent behaviors are willing to learn and stop perpetuating the cycle of violence. Once their experiences are validated, and they don't feel directly blamed, they may get involved in projects that recognize their position and even help engage other men. Many men in powerful positions advocate against gender-based violence against women in their personal and professional lives. This is a significant influence on other men to join the effort.

The Need for Change in Viewing Masculinities

The research has documented and revealed the effects, expressions, and legal and criminal issues related to gender-based violence against women, but there should be more work done to include men in this effort. For example, in El Salvador, a few organizations joined together to campaign against gender-based violence (Bird *et al.*, 2007). One important organization doing this critical work was Centro Bartolomé de las Casas (CBC). The center created a masculinities program to prevent and reduce risk factors impacting gender-based violence and to transform cultural standards that endure or justify violence. This effort was based on the idea that since men need to strive to change their own patterns of behaviors, they need to be taught how to nurture a profound lifelong change. Thus, the CBC program persuades men to model gender-sensitive behavior and inspires other men to change their behaviors. The center designed various activities, such as consciousness-raising, developing leadership roles, creating resources and procedures for use at the community level, and conducting research on El Salvador's masculinities. The program mainly examined the connection between violence and sexual behaviors. The most critical activities were 'masculinities workshops,' letting men explore and closely examine the profound impact of societal beliefs on gender identity and gender relations. The workshops executed three primary approaches in working with men: (1) establishing an atmosphere built on trust and privacy, (2) reconnecting feelings and physiques, and (3) group contemplation and evaluation of the personal and societal meaning of masculinity. All approaches integrate a higher level of emotional understanding using collaborative events and art projects, personal expressions, including reflections and individual and group practices, and debate and evaluation of films, media, and other resources.

It is crucial to blend personal and theoretical analysis when it comes to men's sense of self and relational identity. Many men that were part of the training in El Salvador's CBS program stated that their behavior and outlook changed when the theoretical part of their training was confirmed by everyday interactions and practices in their lives. They learned how to deal with their emotional reactions like confusion, rage, hope, pleasure, and liberation (Bird *et al.*, 2007). The most critical aspects of helping men question their socialization are experiential, emotional, physical, and dynamic learning. They need to be supported to contextualize their gender experience and examine how they are complicit and participate in acts of violence or remain silent when others use violence to solve problems. Men have way fewer opportunities to express their deepest feelings, are constrained by the male gender stereotype, and are expected to be physically and emotionally powerful, intelligent, and treat women as their possessions. Hence, their insecurities need to be validated and supported so that they can adopt a new mindset about what it means to be a man both at home and in society beyond seeing masculinity as possessive, violent, and self-centered. However, this transformation process causes tension between men and other male family members and co-workers who support masculine stereotypes. Thus, emancipated men should build better alliances with other men in preventing gender-based violence and be active agents of change. Religious and community leaders should also be trained to support women's organizations against gender-based violence, help men with their advocacy efforts, and increase women's empowerment by providing funding and helping them with their leadership efforts in public spaces.

The Healing Power of Psychotherapy

Over the years, there have been different schools of thought about the nature of gender-based violence, ranging from the assumption that the male perpetrator or the female victim were dealing with mental health problems and somehow instigated violence to the perception that the violence was somehow liked and stimulated by both partners (Roddy, 2013). We now know that gendered-base violence has many reasons and can be prevented. We are also able to recognize that domestic violence is perpetrated and suffered by men and women (Smith *et al.*, 2018). Cross-culturally, the existence of this kind of violence is no longer excused or has been assumed to be unavoidable. The psychotherapy that is needed for the victims of violence requires a strong bond between the therapist and the client and support and understanding of their unique situation as opposed to a blanket model used for domestic violence (Roddy, 2013).

The models that have been shown to have better efficacy include being nonjudgmental in psychodynamic therapy, having empathy in cognitive behavioral therapy, and unconditional positive regards from the Rogerian therapy model. However, even though external validation, being nonjudgmental, having empathy, and having positive regard for the client are all critical for effective therapy, the long-term psychological impact of abuse and mental health symptoms have to be closely examined and processed. Clients need to hear from the psychotherapist that they did suffer from abuse and did not deserve to suffer using external validation. Furthermore, psychotherapists working with victims of violence must have extensive knowledge about domestic violence, so their issues don't remain unresolved.

Those that have suffered from domestic violence have complex needs and require expert knowledge, longer-term therapy, and lots of unconditional empathy. Given that one in three adults will suffer some form of domestic abuse (Roddy, 2013), psychotherapists need to be familiar with all aspects of the impact of domestic violence. They also have to be willing to be patient with their clients' discovery process. The ending of the therapeutic process has to be decided by the client with the option of coming back if the need arises so there can be a sense of control over decision-making. Overall, a solid therapeutic relationship built on knowledge, trust, and interpersonal dynamics are critical to successful psychotherapy.

Psychotherapy with Male Perpetrators

There are different types of intervention approaches for male perpetrators of domestic violence. The efficacy of these approaches depends on how they get utilized for working with men's behavioral change process using culturally sensitive models to decrease and eventually stop men's violent behavior. According to Saunders (2008), six primary therapy components can be used for intimate partner violence programs: (1) skill-based education; (2) helping men with conflict resolution and managing anger in intimate relationships; (3) reframing maladaptive thoughts; (4) challenging rigid gender stereotypes that supports male abuse of power contributing to violence against women; (5) interventions that challenge family system dynamics and implicit messages supporting violent behavior; and (6) intervention models focusing on post-trauma symptoms (Lawson *et al.*, 2012). Further, five stages of enhancements in men's behaviors are: motivation to show new behaviors, maintain a balanced lifestyle, improving relational interactions with others, learning beneficial relational skills, and asking for support if needed (Lawson *et al.*, 2012). These intervention approaches help men end the unhealthy gendered power relations and unravel and resolve other related issues to develop a constructive and healthy behavior pattern.

Furthermore, some studies have looked into the additional challenges for offenders who experience discrimination and racism, suggesting culturally sensitive treatments to decrease the negative impacts of these experiences (Almeida & Dolan-Delvecchio, 1999; Williams, 1994; Turhan, 2019; Gondolf & Williams, 2001; Williams, 1992; Williams, 1994). Intimate partner and family violence intervention models mostly use cognitive-behavioral therapy, post-modern feminist therapy, the Duluth model, motivational interviewing, and psychodynamic therapy. The following section describes some of these models in more detail.

Cognitive-behavioral therapy – the CBT model perceives violence as learned behavior and focuses on skills training, including communication and assertiveness training (Aldarondo & Malhotra, 2014). This model also uses anger management methods to teach men to use relaxation exercises, time-outs, and alternatives to problem-solving other than violence (Babcock, Green, & Robie, 2004). This treatment aims to help men change their beliefs, attitudes, and behaviors by focusing on women's rights and healthy intimate relationships. Cognitive-behavioral therapy works with clients who are determined to change, do not have issues relating to others, are willing to change their thinking and behavior patterns, and have preliminary skills to fully immerse in the therapy process (Young, 1999). However, according to Lawson *et al.* (2012), many men do not have this complex level of understanding about their own behavior to change and maintain it based on the CBT treatment.

Cognitive-behavioral therapy focuses on increasing skills to recognize abusive behavior instead of promoting men's motivation to participate in the intervention process. This approach has limited efficacy because men justify their violent behavior based on their exposure to their social environment, such as patriarchal values, masculinity, class, power, and lack of culturally sensitive perspectives (Harne & Radford, 2008). Further, the CBT-based interventions do not consider cultural norms and power dynamics based on violent behavior (Langlands, Ward, & Gilchrist, 2009).

Post-modern feminist therapy – Feminist psychotherapy focuses on several fundamental issues men struggle with. These include not valuing relationships at the level men deserve, not disclosing their fears and insecurities, lack of insight about their behavior, lack of empathy about the impact of their behavior on others, lack of understanding about the importance of intimacy, and lack of communication skills (Bograd, 2013). Feminist psychotherapy's primary goal is to increase men's awareness about gender roles and their understanding of the emotional and behavioral patterns and their abuse of power and control techniques (Healey, Smith, & O'Sullivan, 1999). The most important aspect of this type of psychotherapy is realizing that abusive behavior is fundamentally wrong and not the result of past experiences prior to making a conscious choice not to be violent (Healey *et al.*, 1999). If clients are unwilling to engage in therapeutic activities and take responsibility for their actions, feminist psychotherapy may not be the best choice. In that case, perhaps, trauma-based approaches can improve participants' understanding of the behavior and motivate them to become more engaged in the therapeutic process.

Duluth model – The Duluth model utilizes cognitive-behavioral and feminist therapy approaches and relies on psycho-educational activities to change perpetrators' behavior (Gondolf, 2007; Pence & Paymar, 1993). The goal is to increase men's critical consciousness about the impact of gender norms on their perception of women (Gondolf, 2007). The curriculum focuses on how men learn to control and dominate their partners and use the Power and Control Wheel to challenge men's refusal to believe that their violent behavior against their partners is detrimental (Gondolf, 2007). They concentrate on practical skills to prevent violence, promoting egalitarian relationships. The Duluth model analyzes male abusive behavior based on acceptable norms in male-dominated contexts (Langlands *et al.*, 2009), using theoretical and political lenses from feminist and societal perspectives (Day *et al.*, 2009; Murphy & Eckhardt, 2005). The Power and Control Wheel also focuses on race and ethnicity by concentrating on cultural and ethical dynamic forces impacting violent behavior. However, even though the Duluth model seems to be a little more effective than cognitive-behavioral or feminist approaches alone, there is a great need for more culturally sensitive approaches to working with men in therapy.

Motivational interviewing – This is a strengths-based approach focusing on the whole person, prioritizing safety, education, and then being therapeutic (Simmons & Lehmann, 2009). Since motivational interviewing is a strengths-based model, it helps men who use violence to concentrate on skill-building. Their goal is to provide an empathic setting that lessens men's resistance to change and builds a strong working alliance (Bowen *et al.*, 2018; Simmons & Lehmann, 2009; Lawson *et al.*, 2012). They also help men resolve uncertainty around changing their behavior (Rollnick & Miller, 1995; Murphy & Eckhardt, 2005). Further, it helps clients recognize the link between maladaptive behavior and uncertainty about the need for change, which highly influences men to use violent behaviors (Murphy & Eckhardt, 2005). It is also important to state that the rates of reoffending and leaving the domestic violence interventions programs are high among ethnic minority males, reiterating the existence of systemic racism in all social, political, and health services (Waller, 2016). However, this model uses macro-level interventions considering the person's interaction with their environmental context, experience with the criminal justice system, and clients' strength and untapped resources motivating them to change (Saunders, 2009; Silvergleid & Mankowski, 2006).

Moreover, motivational interviewing has been shown to be useful for ethnic minority men who experience racism and unfair treatment even when they try to trust the system and get the help they desperately need (Gondolf & Williams, 2001). According to Bowen *et al.* (2018), developing therapeutic partnership is crucial at the early phase of gender-based violence interventions. This partnership and healthy alliance motivates clients to take actions and become skillful and hopeful in developing a healthy and respectful intimate relationship

Psychodynamic therapy – The set of interventions this model offers, whether used individually or in the context of group therapy, seeks to alter violent behavior by concentrating on destructive relational communications associated with early childhood attachment (Lawson *et al.*, 2012). The best intervention is to help men uncover their emotional issues related to insecure attachment, mental health disorders, and other interactional and relational issues. It is important to realize that individual psychotherapy can perhaps provide a context for men to avoid responsibility for their violent behavior (Harne & Radford, 2008). However, it can also stress the dynamics of gender-based violence using the role of shame as a significant cause of violent behavior necessitating learning to take responsibility for their actions (Brown, 2004). Couple therapy can be a valuable intervention to enhance partners' healthy interaction and cooperation skills once the perpetrator learns to take responsibility for the violent behavior. Family therapy can also be a beneficial intervention for the entire family to learn different ways of relating to each other.

Moreover, men's sense of powerlessness is often linked to their previous experiences with lack of financial resources and emotional and behavioral problems (Adams, 2012). Research shows that when men deal with other relational, personal, and psychological issues such as addictions and high levels of stress-related life events, the intervention for gender-based violence becomes even more challenging (Roy *et al.*, 2013). For ethnic minorities, extra stressors related to migration may create another set of difficulties preventing them from focusing on the anti-violence treatment (Gondolf & Williams, 2001; Hancock & Siu, 2009).

Subsequently, a comprehensive intervention plan must consider helping men resolve psychological and societal issues related to using violence. The help-seeking behavior of some ethnic minorities is impacted by many ecological factors related to their pre-immigration experiences, economic status, gender dynamics in the family, education, their sense of cultural identity, and lower level of acculturation (Almeida & Dolan-Delvecchio, 1999; Kienzler, Spence, & Wenzel, 2019). Many intimate partner violence programs either disregard or dismiss the value that can be added by considering the power of cultural sensitivity (Almeida & Dolan-Delvecchio, 1999). Jayasundara *et al.* (2014) revealed that negative stereotyping, strong patriarchal perspective, religion, and stressors related to the immigration process relate to a perpetuating cycle of violence. Psychotherapists must consider painful experiences of discrimination and oppression and the impact of immigration and the generational family process. Perhaps, some of the most critical deterrence to gender-based violence is offering culturally accurate and sensitive information to support therapeutic recovery and healing that influence perpetrators' positive behavior. For example, many misunderstandings about Islam and Arab cultures are reinforced by media and politicians that paint a picture of Muslim men as inherently aggressive and even violent towards women. This prejudicial perception has heightened the unfair treatment of Muslim men in agencies like the police or social services. Thus, psychotherapists must process the racism and discrimination clients have experienced using multiculturally sensitive approaches in order to build partnership and trust.

Some obstacles to intervention with ethnic minorities are language proficiency, family dynamics, and perhaps even the cultural norms related to the perception of violence. Since many ethnic minorities are not familiar with the therapy process and have difficulties with acculturation due to the host culture's resistance to accepting them, social support systems can be great sources for a positive behavioral change process. Another valuable way to support ethnic minority men to stop abusive behavior is community-based intervention approaches such as recruiting religious leaders in the community to educate, support and protect women and children (Al-Aman, 2012; Kim, 2010). The field of psychotherapy has not been able to develop models that can pay close attention to concerns, dilemmas, and challenges ethnic minority men face when it comes to gender-based violence. The framework has to be based on mutual listening, respect, honoring dignity, and learning from these men's experiences before helping them make better relational decisions (Cemlyn & Allen, 2016). Psychotherapists must be aware of the stigma associated with seeking help and becoming vulnerable. Several research studies show that paying attention to men's participation anxiety is linked to accepting more therapeutic support (Hong & Ku, 2017; Sparrow *et al.*, 2017). Building trust based on understanding clients' cultural, religious, and societal context is vital in how they experience the intervention (Carbajosa *et al.*, 2017; Lomo *et al.*, 2016; McKenzie-Mavinga, 2009). In a study by Turhan (2019) about Turkish men residing in the UK, the participants were afraid of going to prison and never seeing their children again. Their participation in psychotherapy was not voluntary. Psychotherapists working with this group used empathic listening to validate their fears and decrease the attrition rate. It also helped these men understand gender power dynamics and take responsibility for their behaviors. Therefore, experts' awareness of the men's cultural backgrounds, their complicated immigration histories, and lack of understanding of the laws of the host culture should help psychotherapists have more empathy instead of the use of stereotypes and generalizations. Even untrained interpreters or family members to translate have been linked to poor therapeutic outcomes (Pazos & Nadkarni, 2010). The use of trained and professional interpreters has increased the success of gender-based violence interventions for ethnic communities. According to Girishkumar (2014), if we consider violence against women a human rights issue rather than a cultural phenomenon, we will have a much higher success rate with interventions. Further, when perpetrators have experienced childhood trauma or inadequate attachments, a strong therapeutic relationship can be the most influential factor for positive outcomes (Lawson *et al.*, 2012; Taft & Murphy, 2007; Walling *et al.*, 2012). Generally, motivational interviewing and culturally sensitive strategies appear to be more beneficial than cognitive-behavioral therapy.

Psychotherapy with LGBTQT Community

Some data reveal that same-sex couples may experience violence in their intimate relationship at the same rate as heterosexual couples (Mason *et al.*, 2014; Walters *et al.*, 2013). The Center for Disease Control and Prevention report (CDC) by Walters *et al.*, (2013) revealed that 43.8 percent of lesbians, 61.1 percent of bisexual women, and 35 percent of heterosexual women reported being victimized by a partner in their lifetime. Eighty-nine percent of bisexual and 89.5 percent of heterosexual women stated that the perpetrator was a man, while 67.4 percent of lesbians reported only female perpetrators. Furthermore, about 26 percent of gay men, 37.3 percent of bisexual men, and 29 percent of heterosexual men have experienced sexual and physical violence (Walters *et al.*, 2013; Hellemans *et al.*, 2015). Of gay men who have experienced gender-based violence, 90.7 percent were abused by only male perpetrators, and 78.5 percent of bisexual men and 99.5 percent of heterosexual men stated that females were the perpetrators (Walters *et al.*, 2013). There is more scare data on the pervasiveness of partner abuse in transgender relationships. National surveys must collect data on transgender and genderqueer relationships to understand better the relational challenges they face.

Since states set standards and control the intervention programs, in their review of state BIP (Baterer Intervention Program) standards in 42 states, Kernsmith and Kernsmith (2009) found that 51 percent of the regulation presumed men were often the perpetrators of gender-based violence against women. These regulations are based on a heteronormative prejudice, assuming that the men are perpetrators and women are victims. This dichotomous and linear assumption creates problems for treating male perpetrators with male victims and female perpetrators with female victims (Cannon & Buttell, 2015).

Psychotherapists and researchers suggest that particular issues encountered by LGBTQT communities require different kinds of intervention, consisting of LGBTQT-explicit groups and programs to help with their specific needs. These programs must help this population process trauma related to the family of origin, experiences with homophobia, and concerns related to their safety (Cannon *et al.*, 2016). More psychotherapists identifying as LGBTQT can help this population with specific knowledge about sexual minority subgroups to provide more congruent treatment options (Cannon *et al.*, 2016). LGBTQT community centers can also provide awareness about the struggles, problems, and fears LGBTQT people may encounter to help psychotherapists better serve this population (Coleman, 2003).

Psychotherapists need to know the LGBTQT's unique characteristics and forms of abuse, such as homophobia and family rejection, to motivate sexual and gender minority populations to change their perception and behavior (Coleman, 2003). Since the prevalence of gender-based violence, substance abuse, stigmatization, and discrimination in LGBTQT relationships are high (Klostermann *et al.*, 2011; Lewis *et al.*, 2012; Lewis *et al.*, 2017), interventions must pay close attention to the reason and consequences of gender-based violence as well as co-morbidity with other mental health symptoms (Cannon, 2019).

There is a great need for a different set of theory-based interventions beyond the feminist and Duluth model (Ferreira & Buttell, 2016; Ferreira *et al.*, 2017). Incorporating psychodynamic approaches focusing on clients' values and perception, behavioral deficits, trauma, or using psychopathology may be more effective treatments for sex and gender minority perpetrators (Eckhardt *et al.*, 2013; Ferreira & Buttell, 2016). There is also a great need to create specific treatment programs to process experiences of LGBTQT-identified people and educate them about not using violence as the only strategy to deal with conflict in relationships. According to Gondolf (2004), the Alcoholics Anonymous (AA) incorporating batterer intervention approaches can be very helpful for struggling with chemical dependency and violence. Further, LGBTQT centers can offer individual, couples, family, and group therapy for LGBTQT couples and link perpetrators and victims with other resources such as LGBTQT-specific legal services, LGBTQT-sensitive shelters, and court-approved batterer intervention programs.

More researchers and practitioners recommend integrating anti-homophobia, anti-transphobia, anti-colonialism, anti-sexism, and anti-racism programs with gender-based violence interventions. Incorporating these perspectives can lessen the utilization of violence by changing mindsets and behaviors. This paradigm shift helps lift the burden of continuous and painful adaptation from the shoulders of marginalized communities and provides a transformative experience for all clients. There is an abundance of knowledge about the treatment of relational violence. If psychotherapists want to increase the impact of treatment for LGBTQT abusers of gender-based violence, they must generate relevant and focused knowledge and resources across the field.

Conclusion

Gender-based violence intervention methods strive to stop men's aggressive and forceful behavior toward their partners and children. However, each perpetrator's unique experience and circumstances should be considered based on their social, ethnic, class, and cultural backgrounds. Psychotherapists need to be aware of contextual factors in these men's lives and use them appropriately. There has to be straightforward cooperation and collaboration with other services helping men with other issues in their personal lives. It is utterly important to build trustworthy and meaningful relationships with these men and understand the oppression they have experienced themselves.

Racism and prejudice are real challenges, and interventions cannot be successful without considering the impact of these societal challenges. There has to be a serious consideration for their immigration history that impacts their sense of helplessness in the host culture. Some of these men need extra services to heal them from the trauma they have experienced, as well as their psychiatric history and substance abuse. Particularly, understanding perpetrators' difficulties like lack of language proficiency, cultural background, their experiences of racism and discrimination can be instrumental in accessing proper services that impact violent and abusive behavior towards their partners and children. Culturally skilled methods have been identified as the most helpful model for men, women, and LGBTQT populations to help them develop a more considerate and healthy intimate relationship.

References

Adams, P. J. (2012). Interventions with men who are violent to their partners: Strategies for early engagement. *Journal of Marital and Family Therapy, 38*(3), 458–470. https://doi.org/10.1111/j.1752-0606.2012.00320.x.

Aman, A. L. (2012). *Al-Aman evaluation 2008–2012*. https://www.dvip.org/wp-content/uploads/2018/12/Al-Aman-Evaluation-Report.pdf.

Aldarondo, E., & Malhotra, K. (2014). Domestic violence: What every multicultural clinician should know. In M. L. Miville & A. D. Ferguson (Eds.), *Handbook of Race, Ethnicity and Gender in Psychology* (pp. 379–405). (1st ed.). New York: Springer Science & Business Media.

Almeida, R. V., & Dolan-Delvecchio, K. (1999). Addressing culture in batterers intervention. *Violence Against Women, 5*(6), 654–683.

Babcock, J. C., Green, C. E., & Robie, C. (2004). Does batterers' treatment work? A meta-analytic review of domestic violence treatment. *Clinical Psychology Review, 23*(8), 1023–1053. https://doi.org/10.1016/j.cpr.2002.07.001.https://www.unwomen.org/en/digital-library/publications?f%5b0%5d=published_by:2215

Bird, S., Delgado, R., Madrigal, L., Ochoa, J. B., & Tejeda, W. (2007). Constructing an alternative masculine identity: the experience of the Centro Bartolomé de las Casas and Oxfam America in El Salvador. *Gender & Development, 15*(1), 111–121.

Bograd, M. L. (2013). *Feminist Approaches for Men in Family Therapy* (2nd ed.). New York: Routledge.

Bowen, E., Walker, K., & Holdsworth, E. (2018). Applying a strengths-based psychoeducational model of rehabilitation to the treatment of intimate partner violence: Program theory and logic model. *International Journal of Offender Therapy and Comparative Criminology, 0*(0), 1–18.

Brown, J. (2004). Shame and domestic violence: Treatment perspectives for perpetrators from self psychology and affect theory. *Sexual and Relationship Therapy, 19*(1), 39–56. https://doi.org/10.1080/14681990410001640826.

Cannon, C. E. B. (2019). What services exist for LGBTQ perpetrators of IPV in batterer intervention programs across North America? A qualitative study. *Partner Abuse, 10*(2), 222–242. https://doi. org/10.1891/1946-6560.10.2.222.

Cannon, C., & Buttell, F. (2015). Illusion of inclusion: The failure of the gender paradigm to account for intimate partner violence in LGBT relationships. *Partner Abuse, 6*(1), 65–77. https://doi.org/10.1891/1946-6560.6.1.65.

Cannon, C., Hamel, J., Buttell, F. P., & Ferreira, R. J. (2016). A survey of domestic violence perpetrator programs in the United States and Canada: Findings and implications for policy and intervention. *Partner Abuse, 7*(3), 226–276. https://doi.org/10.1891/1946-6560.7.3.226.

Cannon, C., Lauve-Moon, K., & Buttell, F. (2015b). Re-theorizing intimate partner violence through post-structural feminism, queer theory, and the sociology of gender. *Social Sciences, 4*, 668–687. https://doi.org/10.3390/socsci4030668.

Carbajosa, P., Catalá-Miñana, A., Lila, M., Gracia, E., & Boira, S. (2017). Responsive versus treatment-resistant perpetrators in batterer intervention programs: Personal characteristics and stages of change. *Psychiatry, Psychology and Law, 24*(6), 1–15. https://doi.org/10.1080/13218719.2017.1347933.

Cemlyn, S., & Allen, D. (2016). Outreach: Care experiences among Gypsy, Travellers and Roma families. In C. Williams & M. J. Graham (Eds), *Social Work in a Diverse Society:. Transformative practice with black and ethnic minority individuals and communities* (pp 161–180). Bristol: Policy Press.

Chynoweth, S. K., & Patrick, E. M (2007). Sexual violence during firewood collection: income-generation as protection in displaced settings. In G. Terry & J. Hoare (Eds), *Gender-Based Violence* (pp.161–181). Bristol: Oxfam and Chicago: Policy Press.

Coleman, V. E. (2003). Treating the lesbian batterer: Theoretical and clinical considerations—A contemporary psychoanalytic perspective. In D. Dutton & D. J. Sonkin (Eds), *Intimate Violence: Contemporary Treatment Innovations* (pp. 159–206). Binghampton, NY: Haworth Maltreatment & Trauma Press.

Day, A., Chung, D., O'Leary, P., & Carson, E. (2009). Programs for men who perpetrate domestic violence: An examination of the issues underlying the effectiveness of intervention programs. *Journal of Family Violence, 24*(3), 203–212. https://doi.org/10.1007/s10896-008-9221-4.

Eckhardt, C. I., Murphy, C. M.,Whitaker, D. J., Sprunger, J., Dykstra, R., & Woodard, K. (2013). The effectiveness of intervention programs for perpetrators and victims of intimate partner violence. *Partner Abuse, 4*(2), 196–231. https://doi.org/10.1891/1946-6560.4.2.196.

Ferreira, R. J., & Buttell, F. P. (2016). Can a "psychosocial model" help explain violence perpetrated by female batterers?. *Research on Social Work Practice, 26*(4), 362–371. https://doi.org/10.1177/1049731514543665.

Ferreira, R. J., Lauve-Moon, K., & Cannon, C. (2017). Male batterer parenting attitudes: Investigating differences between African American and Caucasian men. *Research on Social Work Practice, 27*(5), 572–581. https://doi.org/10.1177/104973151 5592382.

Girishkumar, D. (2014). From multi to interculturalism? Domestic violence faced by British South Asian women. *Critical Review, 3*(1), 53–70.

Gondolf, E. W. (2004). Evaluating batterer counseling programs: A difficult task showing some effects and implications. *Aggression and Violent Behavior, 9*(6), 605–631. https://doi.org/10.1016/j.avb.2003.06.001.

Gondolf, E. W. (2007). Theoretical and research support for the Duluth Model: A reply to Dutton and Corvo. *Aggression and Violent Behavior, 12*(6), 644–657. https://doi.org/10.1016/j.avb.2007.03.001.

Gondolf, E. W., & Williams, O. J. (2001). Culturally focused batterer counseling for African American men. *Trauma, Violence, & Abuse, 2*(4), 283–295.

Hancock, T. U., & Siu, K. (2009). A culturally sensitive intervention with domestically violent Latino immigrant men. *Journal of Family Violence, 24*(2), 123–132. https://doi.org/10.1007/s10896-008-9217-0.

Harne, L., & Radford, J. (2008). *Tackling Domestic Violence: Theories, Policies and Practice* (1st ed.). Glasgow: McGraw-Hill International.

Hayes, C. (2007). Tackling violence against women: a worldwide approach. In G. Terry & J. Hoare (Eds), *Gender-Based Violence*. Oxfam GB.

Healey, K., Smith, S., & O'Sulivan, C. (1999). *Batterer Intervention: Program Approaches & Criminal Justice Strategies*. Washington, DC: US Department of Justice Office of Justice Programmes, National Institute of Justice.

Hellemans, S., Loeys, T., Buysse, A., Dewaele, A., & De Smet, O. (2015). Intimate partner violence victimization among non-heterosexuals: Prevalence and associations with mental and sexual wellbeing. *Journal of Family Violence, 30*(2), 171–188. https://doi.org/10.1007/s10896-015-9669-y.

Hong, R.-M., & Ku, Y.-H. (2017). Exploring stigma experiences using group therapy amongst people living with schizophrenia in a psychiatric day care center. *Neuropsychiatry, 7*(6), 691–699. https://doi.org/10.4172/Neuropsychiatry.1000266.

Human Rights Watch World Report 2002: Special Issues and Campaigns: HIV/AIDS And Human Rights (hrw.org)

Jayasundara, D., Nedegaard, R., Sharma, B., & Flanagan, K. (2014). Intimate partner violence in Muslim communities. *Art and Social Science Journal, 1,* 2–8. https://doi.org/10.4172/2151-6200.S1-003.

Kernsmith, P., & Kernsmith, R. (2009). Treating female perpetrators: State standards for batterer intervention services. *Social Work, 54*(4), 341–349. https://doi.org/10.1093/sw/54.4.341.https://doi.org/10.1016/j.avb.2011.01.002.

Kienzler, H., Spence, C., & Wenzel, T. (2019). A culture-sensitive and person-centred approach: Understanding and evaluating cultural factors, social background and history when working with refugees. In T. Wenzel & B. Drožđek (Eds.), *An Uncertain Safety* (pp. 101–116). https://doi.org/10.1007/978-3-319-72914-5_5.

Kim, M. (2010). Alternative interventions to intimate violence: defining political and pragmatic challenges. In J. Ptacek (Ed.). *Restorative Justice and Violence against Women* (pp. 193–218). Oxford/New York: Oxford University Press.

Kirk, J. (2007). Gender-based violence in and around schools in conflict and humanitarian contexts. In G. Terry & J. Hoare (Eds), *Gender-Based Violence.* Oxfam, GB

Klostermann, K., Kelley, M. L., Milletich, R. J., & Mignone, T. (2011). Alcoholism and partner aggression among gay and lesbian couples. *Aggression and Violent Behavior, 16*(2), 115–119.

Langlands, R. L., Ward, T., & Gilchrist, E. (2009). Applying the good lives model to male perpetrators of domestic violence. *Behaviour Change, 26*(2), 113–129. https://doi.org/10.1375/bech.26.2.113.

Lawson, D. M., Kellam, M., Quinn, J., & Malnar, S. G. (2012). Integrated cognitive-behavioral and psychodynamic psychotherapy for intimate partner violent men. *Psychotherapy, 49*(2), 190–201. https://doi.org/10.1037/a0028255.

Leach, F., and Humphreys, S. (2007). Gender violence in schools: taking the 'girls-as-victims' discourse forward. In G. Terry & J. Hoare (Eds), *Gender-Based Violence.* Oxfam, GB.

Lewis, R. J., Mason, T. B., Winstead, B. A., & Kelley, M. L. (2017). Empirical investigation of a model of sexual minority specific and general risk factors for intimate partner violence among lesbian women. *Psychology of Violence, 7*(1), 110–119. https://doi.org/10.1037/vio0000036.

Lewis, R. J., Milletich, R. J., Kelley, M. L., & Woody, A. (2012). Minority stress, substance use, and intimate partner violence among sexual minority women. *Aggression and Violent Behavior, 17*(3), 247–256. https://doi.org/10.1016/j.avb.2012.02.004.

Lomo, B., Haavind, H., & Tjersland, O. A. (2016). From resistance to invitations: How men voluntarily in therapy for intimate partner violence may contribute to the development of a working alliance. *Journal of Interpersonal Violence, 33*(16), 1–23. https://doi.org/10.1177/0886260516628290.

Mason, T. B., Lewis, R. J., Milletich, R. J., Kelley, M. L., Minifie, J. B., & Derlega, V. J. (2014). Psychological aggression in lesbian, gay, and bisexual individuals' intimate relationships: A review of prevalence, correlates, and measurement issues. *Aggression and Violent Behavior, 19*(3), 219–234. https://doi.org/10.1016/j.avb.2014.04.001.

McKenzie-Mavinga, I. (2009). *Black Issues in the Therapeutic Process.* Basingstoke, Hampshire: Palgrave Macmillan.

Mehta, M. (2004). Towards ending violence against women in South Asia. Oxfam International.

Murphy, C. M., & Eckhardt, C. I. (2005). *Treating the Abusive Partner: An Individualized Cognitive-behavioral Approach.* New York: Guilford Press.

Pazos, H., & Nadkarni, L. I. (2010). Competency with linguistically diverse population. In J. A. Erickson Cornish (Ed.), *Handbook of Multicultural Counseling Competencies* (pp. 153–195). Hoboken, NJ: John Wiley & Sons.

Pence, E., & Paymar, M. (1993). *Education Groups for Men who Batter: The Duluth model*. New York: Springer Publishing Company.

Reuters Foundation (2005). Uganda: Rape Rampant in Largest Northern IDP Camp. http://www.alertnet.org/thenews/newsdesk.

Roddy, J. K. (2013). Client perspectives: The therapeutic challenge of domestic violence counseling – a pilot study. *Counseling and Psychotherapy Research, 13*(1), 53–60. http://dx.doi.org/10.1080/14733145.2012.711340

Rollnick, S., & Miller, W. R. (1995). What is motivational interviewing? *Behavioural and Cognitive Psychotherapy, 23*(4), 325–334.

Roy, V., Châteauvert, J., & Richard, M.-C. (2013). An ecological examination of factors influencing men's engagement in intimate partner violence groups. *Journal of Interpersonal Violence, 28*(9), 1798–1816. https://doi.org/10.1177/088626051 2469110.

Saunders, D. G. (2009). 8. Programs for men who batter. In E. Stark & E. S. Buzawa (Eds), *Violence Against Women in Families and Relationships [3 volumes]* (3rd ed.) (pp. 161–178). Prager: ABC-CLIO.

Saunders, D. G. (2008). Group interventions for men who batter: A summary of program descriptions and research. *Violence and Victims, 23*(2), 156–172. https://doi.org/10.1891/0886-6708.23.2.156.

Sen, A. (1999). *Development as Freedom*. Oxford: Oxford University Press.

Silvergleid, C. S., & Mankowski, E. S. (2006). How batterer intervention programs work: Participant and facilitator accounts of processes of change. *Journal of Interpersonal Violence, 21*(1), 139–159. https://doi.org/10.1177/0886260505282103.

Simmons, C., & Lehmann, P. (2009). Strengths-based batterer intervention: A new direction with a different paradigm. In P. Lehmann & C. Simmons (Eds), *Strengths-based Batterer Intervention: A New Paradigm in Ending Family Violence* (pp. 39–43). New York: Springer Publishing Company.

Smith, S. G., Zhang, X., Basile, K. C., Merrick, M. T., Wang, J., Kresnow, M., & Chen, J. (2018). *The National Intimate Partner and Sexual Violence Survey (NISVS): 2015 data brief—updated release*. Atlanta, GA: National Center for Injury Prevention and Control, Centers for Disease Control and Prevention.

Sparrow, K., Kwan, J., Howard, L., Fear, N., & MacManus, D. (2017). Systematic review of mental health disorders and intimate partner violence victimisation among military populations. *Social Psychiatry and Psychiatric Epidemiology, 52*(9), 1059–1080. https://doi.org/10.1007/s00127-017-1423-8

Taft, C. T., & Murphy, C. M. (2007). The working alliance in intervention for partner violence perpetrators: Recent research and theory. *Journal of Family Violence, 22*(1), 11–18. https://doi.org/10.1007/s10896-006-9053-z.

Turhan, Z. (2019). *The Lived Experiences of Turkish Perpetrators' Engagement in Domestic Violence Interventions*. London: Goldsmiths, University of London.

United Nations. (1993). *Declaration on the Elimination of Violence against Women*. New York: UN General Assembly. Scientific research publishing. (n.d.). https://www.scirp.org/reference/referencespapers.aspx referenceid=1800452

United Nations. (2006). *The Due Diligence Standard as a Tool for the Elimination of Violence against Women: Report of the Special Rapporteur on violence against women, its causes and consequences*. http://www.un.org/events/res_1325e.pdf

United Nations Economic and Social Council Commission on Human Rights. (2003). *Towards an Effective Implementation of International Norms to End Violence against Women.* http://www.un.org/womenwatch/daw/beijing/platform/plat1.htm.

United Nation Security Council. (2000). https://documents-dds-ny.un.org/doc/ UNDOC/GEN/N00/720/18/PDF/N0072018.pdf?OpenElement/

Waller, B. (2016). Aggression and violent behavior broken fixes: A systematic analysis of the effectiveness of modern and post-modern interventions utilized to decrease IPV perpetration among black males remanded to treatment. *Aggression and Violent Behavior, 27,* 42–49. https://doi.org/10.1016/j.avb.2016.02.003.

Walling, S. M., Suvak, M. K., Howard, J. M., Taft, C. T., & Murphy, C. M. (2012). Race/ethnicity as a predictor of change in working alliance during cognitive behavioral therapy for intimate partner violence perpetrators. *Psychotherapy,* 49(2), 180–189. https://doi.org/10.1037/a0025751.

Walters, M. L., Chen, J. & Breiding, M. J. (2013). *The National Intimate Partner and Sexual Violence Survey (NISVS): 2010 findings on victimization by sexual orientation.* Atlanta, GA: National Center for Injury Prevention and Control, Centers for Disease Control and Prevention.

Williams, O. J. (1992). Ethnically sensitive practice to enhance treatment participation of African American men who batter. *The Journal of Contemporary Human Services, 73*(10), 588–595.

Williams, O. J. (1994). Group work with African American men who batter: Toward more ethnically sensitive practice. *Journal of Comparative Family Studies, 25*(1), 91–103.

World Health Organization. (2005). *Multi-country Study on Women's Health and Domestic Violence against Women.* http://www.who.int/gender/violence/who_multicountry_st udy/summary_report/en/index.html.

World Health Organization. (2021). *Violence Against Women.* https://www.who.int/news-room/fact-sheets/detail/violence-against-women

Young, J. E. (1999). *Cognitive Therapy for Personality Disorders: A Schema-focused Approach.* Professional Resource Press/Professional Resource Exchange.

10 Gender and Work

Introduction

Globally, achieving a proper balance between work and family life is a challenging dilemma all workers encounter. It is critical for the entire family's well-being to balance work, family obligations, and personal life effectively. If more countries develop policies promoting supportive and flexible working contexts, parents can better balance work and home life. Several issues impacting the work and family balance, including working hours, personal care time, and the gender gap in pay, will be discussed below.

Working hours – Part of the work and life balance depends on the number of hours someone is away from home and is working. Research suggests that the length of time we spend at work can influence our well-being, threaten our sense of security, and raise our stress level. According to the Organisation for Economic Co-operation and Development (OECD), in 2014, globally, 11 percent of employees worked 50 or more hours weekly. This report reveals that 33 percent of workers in Turkey are working very long hours. Mexico, with about 29 percent, and Colombia, with close to 27 percent of employees, are among the countries with the highest working hours. The OECD data (2014) shows that men work longer hours with over 15 percent, compared with about 6 percent for women.

Personal care – Longer work hours leave less time for other activities, like self-care or leisure. Our overall physical well-being and mental health improve with quality leisure time. According to OECD data, a full-time worker dedicates 63 percent or 15 hours of any given day for personal care such as eating, sleeping, socializing with friends and family, relaxing, and using media for entertainment. It is interesting that even though women may not work as many hours as men, they still don't have more leisure time, and their self-care time is the same as for the men across the 20 OECD countries.

Gender gap in pay – The gender gap in pay in the US has continued to stay the same for the past 15 years. According to the Pew Research Center findings, based on the median hourly earnings of both full- and part-time workers, women's income was 84 percent of men's earnings, equal to an extra 42 days of work for women. An analysis of full-time workers by the US Census Bureau

DOI: 10.4324/9781003088189-11

reveals that in 2019, women's income was 82 percent of men's earnings (Semega *et al.*, 2020). It is possible to measure the gap by considering education, types of occupation, and the number of years in the workforce. Even though women have been getting an education at a higher rate and are more represented in higher-paying jobs like specialized and managerial positions, women continue to be overrepresented in lower-paying jobs compared to their workforce presence. Thus, gender discrimination can be one of the main contributors to the continuing wage difference. Pew Research in 2017 showed that approximately 42 percent of working women state that they experienced gender discrimination at work, but only 22 percent of men state that they had the same experience (Parker & Funk, 2017). The most cited type of discrimination was earning disparity, with 25 percent of women earning less than a man who performed the exact same job, while only 5 percent of men had the same claim.

Another factor that impacted women more than men was motherhood, interrupting women's career paths and their long-term income (Gangl & Ziefle, 2009). Pew Research in 2016 found that women take more time off (closer to 11 weeks) than men (one week) after giving birth or adopting a child (Horowitz *et al.*, 2017). Over half of women surveyed took more than 12 weeks and stated that the time off impacted their careers. Women's challenges related to juggling caregiving duties and working also add to their stress since they tend to take on more household tasks than their fathers. Mothers with children often reduce their work hours or turn down a promotion to care for their families. About 25 percent of mothers felt that they did not get a promotion or were assigned to important positions, and 27 percent stated that their level of commitment to work was questioned (Semega *et al.*, 2020).

Triple Thread of Work, Family, and Personal Life

Globally work-life has consumed most of our lives, contributing to more work-life imbalance, higher work-family conflicts, and much more stress. Breaks from work are briefer, and vacations are often interrupted by work. The internet and social media are also impeding our quality family time. Consequently, 75–90 percent of doctors' visits are stress-related health issues. According to Davidson *et al.* (2010), stress is associated with the six leading causes of death: heart disease, cancer, lung diseases, accidents, liver disease, and suicide. Stress also influences family relationships and can be passed around to other family members, co-workers, friends, and even the community at large (Moen *et al.*, 2015).

The best model used for an ideal employee is based on a male model of work who works full-time and is fully devoted to his job from the time he gets hired until he retires (Lewis, 1997). This model has created strong burdens, stress, job dissatisfaction, work-family imbalance, and time famine for workers (Greenhaus & Beutell, 1985; Kossek & Lambert, 2005). Further, this model is not relevant anymore since the newer generations do not perceive career success based on these parameters. They are more innovative about quality of work, the definition of commitment, and advancing in their careers. They strive for a better balance for both highly successful professional and personal lives. It makes total sense that organizations that value balancing work and life have a higher chance of attracting talented and highly skilled workers.

Shifting Demographics

Across the world, women have been participating in paid work, and consequently, dual-income families have grown, creating a shift in role expectations, both at home and work (Bond *et al.*, 1998). The higher level of women's participation in the labor force has many encouraging impacts, such as the rise of productivity, family prosperity, women's financial independence, and the enhancement of gender equality. There are also some discouraging pressures on the family in shifting role expectations, insufficient family time, and finding innovative behaviors to balance professional and personal lives. Highly educated professionals tend to get a better sense of identity from their careers than family life and perhaps perceive children as distractions to their productivity. Working women also tend to delay pregnancy and choose to have children later, impacting their fertility. In other words, changes in workplace demographics may have created the potential for a strain on work and life balance and burnout. Some of these changes in the family structure are fully reflected by the national consensus data. In the 1981 census, the population grew faster than households. In the 1991 census, there was a reversal in trend, showing households grew at a faster rate than the population and became a more significant phenomenon after 2000, indicating growth in nuclearization of families.

Culture and Work-Family Balance

The perception of career success and life balance varies in different cultures. One of the additional challenges hard to overcome is cultural norms prioritizing work over family (Lewis, 1997). For example, the capitalistic system of the US creates a context for more people prioritizing money and careers, working on weekends, and taking shorter and fewer breaks from their jobs. Most Western societies do a better job in having a firmer boundary around personal and professional life, preferring more extended vacations to extra pay at work. For example, the Netherlands has the lowest average annual working hours of 35 hours per week for 39 weeks (Jacobs & Gornick, 2001).

On the other hand, people living in developing countries like Turkey, Mexico, Columbia, and India require people to work more hours than people living in some Western countries. Furthermore, due to the surge of technology, the work culture has changed globally over the past few decades. It has pressured us to work faster and accomplish more tasks from anywhere and at any time, potentially interrupting our family time as well as our personal time.

Gender Equality and Work

Extensive research shows that psychological and contextual stressors of work impact the quality of our personal lives, forming work-family conflict (WFC) (Ammons & Kelly, 2015; Gangl *et al.*, 2009; French *et al.*, 2017; Lapierre *et al.*, 2017; Wayne *et al.*, 2017). Work-family conflict influences our health and life quality, impacting work performance and fulfillment, adding to the conflictual relationships at home, and decreasing family satisfaction. Since gender equality at home affects our gender equality at work, the inadequate participation in family responsibilities between men and women is connected to higher work-family conflicts for women.

Thus, understating the impact of gender roles on work conflict is highly critical since the identified sex of the family member primarily determines the foundation for the separation of tasks between men and women in most societies (Wood & Eagly, 2010). In Western cultures, empirical research shows that women are primarily in charge of household tasks creating role strains. The same pattern exists in most nations worldwide. Meta-analyses by different researchers (Byron, 2005; Eby *et al.*, 2005) have confirmed the crucial impact of gender, constantly finding differences in work-home conflict for women and men. These gender role expectations and gender role ideologies are mainly based on mainstream cultural socialization that continuously gets recreated by men and women.

Further, this critical social discourse focuses on the crucial and differing aspects of men's and women's strengths and traits, completely disregarding the social and political contextual factors. It states that men and women make conscious choices based on their natural abilities leading to more women wanting to stay home and more men wanting to work outside of the home (Kuo *et al.*, 2018). This traditional gender role perspective assumes that it is more important for men to have instrumental roles and work outside the home. At the same time, it is more important for women to care for the family and handle the expressiveness aspects of their families (Parsons & Bales, 1955). The traditional gender role model separates the expressiveness axis for men from the instrumentality axis for women under the assumption that these two are distinct and mutually exclusive categories. According to Ollier-Malaterre and Foucreault, 2017, the complicated interactions between work and family are rooted in the broader cultural and economic context related to the disparity in gender equality (Lucas-Thompson & Goldberg, 2015). A study by Martínez and Paterna (2009) found that gender ideology directly links the ratio of responsibilities like shopping and preparing food, washing, and cleaning to be traditionally feminine, creating a discrepancy in meaning for men and women. Unfortunately, even recent studies show that labor division is still based on gender but may vary in different households. This means that we need men and women to be instrumental and expressive inside and outside their homes.

Impact of Household Tasks on Work-Family Conflict (WFC)

The relational conflict in families, especially those with children, is partly around the time needed for household responsibilities and caring for the family. Dual-income couples with children struggle more with the stress of balancing work and family than couples without children (Michel & Hargis, 2008).

However, caring for children and household responsibilities have different implications for women than men in many countries (Korabik, 2015; Organization for Economic Cooperation and Development [OECD] 2014; Eurobarometer, 2015). For example, in Spain, every week, women spend almost twice as much time as men on unpaid work in caring for children for about 38 hours versus 23 for men; caring for family members for about 20 hours versus 14 hours for men; and household responsibilities for about 20 hours versus 11 hours for men. Thus, even though more women are now working outside their homes, they are still spending more time taking care of their children and household responsibilities.

On the other hand, most men work full-time without interruption since their partners often undertake the obligation of caring for their children and home. Consequently, women's work life is much more interrupted by family responsibilities because they have less time, concentration, and commitment to their work. On the other hand, men's family life gets more interrupted by work.

Furthermore, men have not been socialized to see the need to take responsibility for household tasks as much as women. At best, men have been socialized to choose to help around the house and need appreciation as a reward. The other challenge for women is that household tasks like cooking and cleaning are daily activities, while men paying bills, taking care of the yard, or fixing the car are not daily tasks. Our cultural socialization has us convinced that women's identity is much more connected to having power in the family realm, and they don't want to give up this power. In contrast, men's sense of gender identity is more linked to paid work, which should be reinforced (Martínez & Paterna, 2009). However, in reality, men's lack of participation with tasks at home and bringing work stress home cause more household responsibilities for women. The stress, then, impacts marital conflicts, which influence women's productivity at work. On the other hand, men's contribution to household tasks does not increase if women have a higher level of work stress. Studies on family relationships reveal that when couples are stressed, they have a higher level of destructive interactions and disagreements. (Westman & Etzion, 2005; Huffman *et al.*, 2017). This harmful interaction results in negative responses, criticism, conflict, and negative marital interactions.

Decision-Making

Traditionally, in a couple's relationship, the balance of power depends on the comparative resources each partner provides. The one contributing more has a more significant influence over the decision-making process. However, research shows that even when couples perceive their relationship as equal, husbands are mostly the decision-maker, contributing to more gender inequality (Fox & Murry, 2000). Husbands use their power to indirectly influence decision-making processes by denying potential conflicts about household tasks (Ball *et al.*, 1995). Social exchange theory suggests that men hold decision-making power because of their access to more economic resources, education, and higher career advancements (Scanzoni, 1982). The conflict theory hypothesizes that relational conflict between husband and wife is related to using power and control over resources using collaboration and conflict management to control the result of the decision-making process (Sprey, 1979), leading to much greater influence over decision making for men. However, for dual-income families, this process may be different. Equality in decision-making by both partners is highly beneficial for relational satisfaction. Nevertheless, even in more modern forms of marriage, decision-making is separated by traditional gender lines. Women are in charge of decision-making for everyday family life, and men are still making critical decisions, like distributing resources.

Gender Role Attitudes

Traditional gender roles determine the areas of expertise for men and women, dictating that men should have power in the outside world, and women should have the power inside the home and be in charge of relationship maintenance. Relational aspects of women's life give them inadequate access to resources outside the home and high levels of relational dependence. On the other hand, men have access to power and status based on their earning ability and are responsible for family monetary resources. This level of power, mixed with their traditional patriarchal status of being the ultimate power, creates a context for men being exempt from everyday responsibilities of a household (Scanzoni, 1982). This unbalanced access to resources contributes to the husband's career being deemed to be of greater value than his wife's career, which elevates his position in all aspects of family life. His work outside the home is considered time spent earning money for the family, granting him less contribution to household tasks. Since the wife's career is not perceived as financially essential, her time at work does not exempt her from gendered household tasks.

Interestingly, even now that 57 percent of women are working (statusofwomendata.org, 2014), the husband's career is still assumed to be more important. The wife's status is considered to have less importance, even when her career has high marketplace value (Steil, 1997). This appraisal of whose career is essential to family life reduces wives' access to vital resources and attributes different weights to contributions by husbands or wives. Even though newer patterns are forming for younger couples, this gender role ideology creates a primary and consistently high level of stress for working couples. The heightened stress level impacts couples when patterns of behavior in the relationship and values about gender equality contradict each other. Though research has shown that couples who believe in relational equality strive to have a more reasonable division of labor (Greenstein, 1996b; Presser, 1994; Sanchez, 1994), actual equality in the dividing household responsibilities is still lacking.

Blair and Johnson (1992) found a modest but considerable association between gender ideology and the distribution of household tasks, indicating that conflict may occur if the division of household tasks goes against one's gender ideology. However, according to Greenstein (1996a), an unequal division of household responsibilities impacts relational quality for wives with non-traditional gender role values instead of wives with more traditional gender role values.

Division of Household Responsibilities

Many studies have documented overwhelming global support for women to engage in career activities and become politically active, advocating for equal gender identity. Even though, ideally, more men have embraced the idea of gender equality, they are still not doing their share of responsibilities at home. Approximately 25 percent of high school seniors asked about their perfect model for home life, preferred an arrangement with fathers working full time and mothers staying home. Young men in heterosexual relationships are no more inclined to do household tasks than the older generation. According to the Organization for Economic Cooperation and Development data, women spend four hours compared to men, who spend 2.5 hours of unpaid work a day.

Furthermore, studies show that dual-earner couples contribute more to household responsibilities than when men are the primary breadwinner (DeMeis & Perkins, 1996; Greenstein, 2000). However, one critical factor is that this perceived shared responsibility may be more related to wives' lower contribution to household tasks and not necessarily higher contribution by men. For instance, research shows that the husband's equal contributions to household tasks fluctuate between 2 percent and 12 percent (Ferree, 1991). The idea of quality and fairness related to the performance of household tasks bothers women more than men because they are more burdened by the tasks than are their husbands, which contributes to a higher level of relational conflict, or women sidestepping the disagreement to lower the marital conflict. The distributive justice framework discussed by Major (1987) states that women's assessment of fairness in the division of household tasks is often based on the societal perception of fairness, valuing men's contribution at a higher level than women's contribution. Women perceive the expected higher contribution to household tasks as compensation for men's financial contributions and their share. Social norms also determine what types of work are women's work and justify the unbalanced distribution of household tasks. Thus, if all husbands are not making an effort to contribute to family life, then women perceive their situation the same as others and as fitting the social norm. The social comparison theory suggests that we evaluate our life situations by comparing them to the life of others. Thus, women were satisfied if compared to other men (friends and family), their husbands did more household tasks, and they were able to do fewer household tasks compared to other women (Himsel & Goldberg, 2003).

Unfair division of household tasks can have a substantial impact on many other aspects of marital relationships, such as depression and marital discord (Coltrane, 2000; Rogers & Amato, 2000), marital unhappiness (Blair, 1998), and discontent (Kluwer *et al.*, 1996, 1997). A study examining dual-career relationships showed an association between the lower level of marital happiness and both husband and wife believing that they do more household tasks than the other (Frisco & Williams, 2003). Further, wives' perceptions about doing more household tasks than their husbands contributed to a higher divorce rate. On the other hand, when partners make joint decisions about the division of tasks, wives' perception of relational equality improves. Better relational patterns emerge when husbands contribute to household tasks at a higher rate as part of this collaborative decision-making. More importantly, when husbands expressed gratitude and concern for their wives' amount of work, wives' perception of equality and fairness improved (Hawkins *et al.*, 1998).

There are low control tasks like the ones women are often in charge of, such as cooking and cleaning, that need to be repeated on a daily basis, and there are high control tasks that men are often in charge of and are not time-dependent. Studies have shown that tasks can impact physical well-being more than the time it may take to finish the task (Barnett & Rivers, 1996; Barnett & Shen, 1997). Low control tasks were often linked to physical symptoms of stress, while high control tasks did not have the same effects. It seems like meeting the needs of family members can be a strong predictor of emotional stress, which often is associated with low control tasks (Barnett & Shen, 1997). The most thought-provoking aspect of this finding is that gender did not have a mediating influence. Thus, men and women equally felt that spending time on low control tasks lowered their marital quality (Barnett & Rivers, 1996); impacted their emotional stress (Barnett & Shen, 1997); heightened their sense of inequality (Sanchez & Kane, 1996), and increased relational conflict (Perry-Jenkins & Folk, 1994).

Relational Justice

The quality of marital relationships significantly improves when partners perceive the costs and benefits of being in a committed relationship are fair, and each partner's contributions are acknowledged. A sense of equality is when partners feel that their investment in the relationship is comparable to the rewards they receive, and no one feels overwhelmed or overworked. The important part of this is that when the family and relational stress is low, the lack of fair distribution of tasks does not significantly contribute to disagreements over tasks. But it becomes a significant source of conflict when the couple's stress level is high and partners feel the other is not carrying the weight. Research has repeatedly shown a correlation between marital satisfaction and just perceiving that the level of contribution is equal. However, many partners who perceive themselves as contributing equally fail to do so. Furthermore, wives who are the primary source of financial support for the family tend to assess their husbands' contribution as not equitable and demand more help (Ferree, 1987).

Couples' relationships are now impacted by women's higher financial contribution and, consequently, the higher demands for equal distributions of household tasks. On the other hand, husbands have always enjoyed the benefits of contributing less and benefiting more from an unequal relationship. They tend to criticize their wives less and are more content with their relationship if their wives do a higher share of the household tasks (Barnett & Baruch, 1987). They also do not perceive their marital satisfaction, personal happiness, and psychological health as depending on the division of household tasks. Thus, couples must move away from the traditional division of household labor, unequal decision-making power, and old-fashioned gender role expectations and move more in the direction of fairness, equality, and egalitarian decision-making, fair perception of each other's contributions, and performing with the definitive level of honor and justice.

Gender, Power, and Financial Resources

There is a strong association between having power and access to financial resources in any relationship globally, except for a marital relationship. Pew Research in 2017 reported that in 28 percent of heterosexual relationships, women earn more money than men. However, women's greater access to financial resources and earning higher incomes have not impacted their decision-making or major financial decisions. Married women with higher income try even harder to make their husbands not feel threatened by their wives' earning power, perpetuating the vicious cycle of gender-based power inequality in their relationship (Atwood, 2012; Knudson-Martin, 2012). In fact, cross-culturally, believing in men's role as providers for the family has been consistently strengthened (Atwood, 2012; Pew Research Center, 2017).

In the US, African Americans, Latinos, and those groups with lower educational attainments are more influenced by this double standard holding men accountable for providing for their families. In their survey, Pew Research Center (2017) found that 84 percent of African Americans and 78 percent of Latino adults considered men good husbands if they provided for their families. On the other hand, 52 percent of African Americans and 40 percent of Latinos believed providers are also good wives. Approximately 81 percent of those with high school or lower education had the same belief. Research shows that men with lower earning power than their wives may struggle with a lower sense of self, depression, and marital conflict because they feel they are not providing for the family at a socially expected level (Atwood, 2012).

Reciprocity in Relationship

Financial resources are a great source of interaction for couples. It can show love and devotion when one spends money on the other partner, and it can define dependency or autonomy based on how money is used for relationship stability (Atwood, 2012). Studies show that discussing finances is a great source of conflict among conflictual topics such as parenting, household tasks, and communication (Papp *et al.*, 2009; Atwood, 2012). A healthy pattern of giving and taking in a stable relationship can be a great asset, even though it can become a rigid model for expectations. For example, the spouse that makes more money may expect a higher level of gratitude and higher contribution to household tasks in exchange for providing stable financial resources. The inflexible expectations for equal exchange impact relationship satisfaction and create conflicts. However, in this exchange of resources, gender is one of the leading contextual factors influencing the give and take process. It is incredibly invisible, concealed, and not even part of couples' conscious relational patterns (Knudson-Martin, 2012). Thus, men's needs become the core of the couples' relationship, shaping their dynamics with men stonewalling to deny the needs of their wives and women silencing themselves to adapt to their husbands' demands (Knudson-Martin, 2012).

The Healing Power of Psychotherapy

Gender equality between men and women can strongly impact the effective management of societies and family and work (Wharton, 2015). Eventually, the societal changes based on gender equality will create a context for both men and women to perceive both work and family environments as necessary and contribute equally to both (Kuo *et al.*, 2018). This does not mean that women will not contribute to family life any less. It simply means men and women can be involved in both without creating much work-family conflict for women (Lucas-Thompson & Goldberg, 2015). Likewise, those specializing in strengthening family life must consider that due to all economic changes globally, men are not able to be the sole breadwinner for the family. Thus, there is a need to homogenize women's and men's family and workplace responsibilities. Work institutions can contribute to this societal change by creating family-friendly policies to strengthen the pursuit of a better home and work balance for both men and women (Lin *et al.*, 2017; Matias *et al.*, 2017). For example, couple and family therapy and premarital training can help couples learn how to coordinate their commitment to the family, decrease work stress, reduce relational conflict, diminish WFC, and balance work and family life. This will significantly enhance the quality of their workers' dedication, which results in a return of investment (ROI) for the organization (Dowd *et al.*, 2017) and make a fundamental contribution to having fairer societies.

According to Knudson-Martin (2012), if cross-culturally, couples understand the gender norms impacting their everyday interactions and avoid it, they can develop more egalitarian relationships. It is also important to become consciously aware of the value of women's work, honor differences, and not get intimidated by other viewpoints impacting their relationship. Couples also need to develop skills to become more effective in conflict management. Additionally, gender role flexibility can significantly contribute to equality in heterosexual couple relationships (Knudson-Martin, 2012). Based on these guidelines, psychotherapists must engage men in developing relational skills to preserve the marital relationship with less dominance and more emotional support for relationship growth instead of holding women responsible for the emotional aspects of the relationship.

The appraisal of couples' level of awareness of the other's emotions and desires, the capacity to allow each other to develop separate interests and activities, and shared activities are all critical for the couples' common welfare (Knudson-Martin, 2012). Knudson-Martin and Mahoney (2009) suggested that in assessing the level of stress couples experience with distribution of money and power inequalities in the relationship, psychotherapists should consider four elements of relational status, consideration of others, accommodating others, and health. Psychotherapists need to observe interactional patterns and ask about the couple's relationship-building skills set. Psychotherapists can also inquire about the importance of the relationship for each partner, their mutual and separate interests, their decision-making process, their contribution to the relationship's emotional health, and their level of interest in the financial well-being of their partner.

Couples' social and cultural context related to norms, roles, and expectations should be the basis of assessing issues related to money and equality in the relationship. When couples better understand the sociopolitical and cultural partners impacting their relationship satisfaction, they become less defensive about their own behavior and are more likely to change. There are times that one partner is from a collectivistic (we pull our resources together) background and the other partner is from an individualistic background (we don't rely on anyone for help). Thus, their personal interests and goals may be completely different from each other without even being conscious of it. Psychotherapists must be able to assess these backgrounds and see how these couples pay attention to the desires and feelings of each other based on their social and cultural backgrounds. Psychotherapists must choose therapeutic interventions based on partners' cultural backgrounds in using direct or indirect communication to discuss finances and to discuss how give and take in a relationship is defined in hierarchical relationships. The developmental stage and life-cycle transitions are essential components impacting relational equality in families. Creating a separate and functional relational system distinct from the family of origin and negotiating different rules and obligations is part of forming a healthy partnership (McGoldrick & Shibusawa, 2012). This means that psychotherapists should help newly married partners negotiate things such as the frequency of seeing friends and families, patterns of saving and spending money and creating healthy boundaries with their families of origin (McGoldrick & Carter, 2003). These negotiations and boundary-making processes are the foundation of egalitarian relationships.

On the other hand, couples that have retired also need to renegotiate plans related to spending money on vacations, having a separate and healthy relationship with children and grandchildren, and perhaps more flexible gender roles to promote relational equality (Bookwala, 2012). According to DeMaris *et al.* (2012), gender equality is directly linked to relationship satisfaction, and lack of equality disturbs relational closeness and positive connections between partners. Therefore, psychotherapists must evaluate patterns of contributions in different aspects of the couple's life, such as household tasks and financial decision-making, to encourage couples to define relational equality. This is only possible when both partners have a good understanding of the power dynamics in their relationship. Couples also need to develop specific behavioral competencies to successfully convey their needs and desires, understand and accept their differences, and learn effective ways to relate to one another. Using systems theory, psychotherapy must provide valuable tools for couples to focus on relational inequality and develop equal and effective partnerships.

One of the crucial elements of systems theory is circular causality signifying the reciprocal dynamics of couples' relations in terms of behaviors, emotions, and thoughts that are impacted by each other and the couples' context. Thus, psychotherapists must pay close attention to emotional and behavioral exchanges in the relationship and consider all environmental, developmental, and personal aspects that influence relational functioning (Baucom *et al.*, 2015). These developmental, ecological, normative, and non-normative challenges such as chronic illness, death in the family, or childbirth require sufficient resources (Dattilio & Epstein, 2016). Psychotherapists must help couples expand their awareness and skills in regulating their intense relational emotions, assess their beliefs about each other's behavioral intentions, and adjust personal actions to increase positive interactions. Further, research reveals that when couples accept each other's differences and use positive communication to convey their perspectives, they have a higher level of relationship adjustment (Fischer *et al.*, 2016). Baucom *et al.* (2015) indicated that when men acknowledge relational challenges and how they may contribute to marital discord, women reported a higher level of marital satisfaction. Psychotherapeutic treatment should begin with a systematic and broad appraisal of each partner's personal attributes such as personality style, mental health issues, desires, ideals, relationship history, and conflict resolution tactics. Any added stressors such as racial and gender discrimination, employment issues, and relationship conflict with extended family members impact financial decision-making and need to be evaluated.

Money is often a proxy for power in most couple relationships, and how couples handle financial concerns is metaphoric for other struggles in sharing resources. It is vital to foster relational equality by resolving role distribution and decision-making disparities. In particular, relational interventions should focus on recognizing partners' beliefs about equality and gender roles and how these beliefs shaped their experience of their interactions. Some examples of how psychotherapists can help increase partners' understanding are reframing men's controlling behavior as working hard to provide for the family and women's complaints about an equal partnership elevating relational satisfaction. It is essential to reframe conflicts about financial resources as a common relational problem in dual-earner families, and having conflicts means mutual engagement, which indicates strong relational bonds. The topic of role distribution and sharing, including budgeting and accounting tasks, is of paramount consideration. Once couples have the realization that sharing is never about having 50/50 distributions of tasks and resources, and it is more about a fair balance of responsibilities, their relational quality will improve.

Conclusion

When individuals have better work and life balance, they experience better health, have a higher sense of commitment, higher job satisfaction, and achieve much higher goals. Further, a healthier work-life balance fosters better relational stability, family unity, and relational contentment. It is crucial for work, family, and personal life to be a source of complement and not conflict with each other. Some people are very successful in their professions and do not succeed in family and personal life. Others have a healthy personal and family life, but they are not thriving in their work environment. If one aspect of life must be sacrificed for another part of life, the result is not relational happiness. A healthy and vibrant personal and family life is a foundation for a successful career in the bigger picture of life. The work and life balance are hardly achievable if we don't try hard, but we can have a much healthier lifestyle if we do try. Psychotherapists need to consider work-life balance as a priority issue to protect the social fabric of societies against permanent destruction.

It is critically important to understand the relational equality in committed relationships, including issues related to financial matters. The cultural and family values and norms that hinder relational equality when negotiating rules, roles, and responsibilities should be considered. It is helpful for psychotherapists to examine how financial resources and gender beliefs learned in families of origin impact gender equality. Couple therapists must also find empirical research to help same-sex couples support the development of equal partnerships (Green, 2012; Moore, 2008).

References

Ammons S. K., & Kelly E. L. (Eds). (2015). *Work and Family in the New Economy. Research in the Sociology of Work* (Vol. 26). Bingley: Emerald Group Publishing Limited. 10.1108/S0277-283320150000026006

Atwood, J. D. (2012). Couples and money: The last taboo. *American Journal of Family Therapy*, *40*, 1–19. http://dx.doi.org/10.1080/01926187.2011.600674

Ball, J., Cowan, P., & Cowan, P. (1995). Who's got the power? Gender differences in partners' perceptions of influence during marital problem-solving discussions. *Family Process, 34*, 303–321.

Barnett, R. C., & Baruch, G. K. (1987). Determinants of fathers' participation in family work. *Journal of Marriage and the Family, 49*, 29–40.

Barnett, R. C., & Rivers, C. (1996). *She Works/He Works: How Two-income Families Are Happier, Healthier, and Better Off.* New York: HarperCollins.

Barnett, R. C., & Shen, Y. C. (1997). Gender, high- and low-schedule control housework tasks, and psychological distress: A study of dual-earner couples. *Journal of Family Issues, 18*, 403–428.

Baucom, D. H., Epstein, N. B., Kirby, J. S., & LaTaillade, J. J. (2015). Cognitive-behavioral couple therapy. In A. S. Gurman, J. L. Lebow, & D. K. Snyder (Eds), *Clinical Handbook of Couple Therapy* (pp. 23–60). New York: Guilford Press.

Blair, S. L. (1998). Work roles, domestic roles, and marital quality: Perceptions of fairness among dual-earner couples. *Social Justice Research, 11*, 313–335.

Blair, S. L. & Johnson, M. P. (1992). Wives' perceptions of the fairness of the division of household labor: The intersection of housework and ideology. *Journal of Marriage and the Family, 54*, 570–771.

Bond, J. T., Galinsky, E., & Swangberg, J. E. (1998). *The 1997 National Study of Changing Workspace.* New York: Families and Work Institute.

Bookwala, J. (2012). Marriage and other partnered relationships in middle and late adulthood. In R. Blieszner & V. Hilkevitch Bedford (Eds), *Handbook of Families and Aging* (2nd ed., pp. 91–123). Santa Barbara, CA: Praeger ABC-CLIO.

Byron, K. (2005). A meta-analytic review of work-family conflict and its antecedents. *Journal of Vocational Behavior, 67*(2) 169–198. http://doi.org/10.1016/j.jvb.2004.08.009

Coltrane, S. (2000). Research on household labor: Modeling and measuring the social embeddedness of routine family work. *Journal of Marriage and the Family, 62*, 1208–1233.

Dattilio, F. M., & Epstein, N. B. (2016). Cognitive-behavioral couple and family therapy. In T. L. Sexton & J. Lebow (Eds), *The Handbook of Family Therapy* (pp. 89–119). New York: Routledge.

Davidson, K.W., Mostofsky, E. & Whang, W. (2010). Don't worry, be happy: Positive affect and reduced 10-year incident coronary heart disease: The Canadian Nova Scotia Health Survey. *European Heart Journal, 31*, 1065–1070.

DeMaris, A., Sanchez, L. A., & Krivickas, K. (2012). Developmental patterns in marital satisfaction: Another look at covenant marriage. *Journal of Marriage and Family, 74*, 989–1004. http://dx.doi.org/10.1111/j.1741-3737.2012.00999.x

DeMeis, D. K. & Perkins, H. W. (1996). "Supermoms" of the nineties: Homemaker and employed mothers' performance and perceptions of the motherhood role. *Journal of Family Issues, 17*(6), 776–792.

Dowd, W. N., Bray, J. W., Barbosa, C., Brockwood, K., Kaiser, D. J., Mills, M. J., ... & Wipfli, B. (2017). Cost and return on investment of a work-family intervention in the extended care industry: evidence from the work, family & health netwrok. *Journal of Occupational and Environmental Medicine, 59*(10), 956. http://doi.org/10.1097/JOM.0000000000001097

Eby, L. T., Casper, W. J., Lockwood, A., Bordeaux, C., & Brinley, A. (2005). Work and family research in IO/OB: content analysis and review of the literature (1980–2002). *Journal of Vocational Behavior, 66*(1), 124–197. http://doi.org/10.1016/j.jvb.2003.11.003

Eurobarometer. (2015). *Gender equality report.* . Retrieed from http://ec.europa.eu/just ice/genderequality/files/documents/eurobarometer_report_2015_en.pdf

Ferree, M. M. (1987). Family and job for working-class women: Gender and class systems seen from below. In N. Gerstel & H. E. Gross (Eds), *Families and Work* (pp. 289–301). Philadelphia, PA: Temple University Press.

Ferree, M. M. (1991). The gender division of labor in two-earner marriages: Dimension of variability and change. *Journal of Family Issues, 12*, 158–180.

Fischer, M. S., Baucom, D. H., & Cohen, M. J. (2016). Cognitive-behavioral couple therapies: Review of the evidence for the treatment of relationship distress, psychopathology, and chronic health conditions. *Family Process, 55*, 423–442. http://dx.doi.org/10.1111/famp.12227

Fox, G. L., & Murry, V. M. (2000). Gender and families: Feminist perspectives and family research. *Journal of Marriage and the Family, 62*, 1160–1172.

French, K. A., Dumani, S., Allen, T. D., & Shockley, K. M. (2017). A meta-analysis of work-family conflict and social support. *Psychological Bulletin, 144*(3), 284. http://doi.org/10.1037/bul0000120

Frisco, M. L., & Williams, K. (2003). Perceived housework equity, marital happiness, and divorce in dual-earner households. *Journal of Family Issues, 24*, 51–73.

Gangl, M., & Ziefle, A. (2009). Motherhood, labor force behavior, and women's Careers: An empirical assessment of the wage penalty for motherhood in Britain, Germany, and the United States. *Demography, 46*(2), 341–369. http://doi.org/10.1353/dem.0.0056

Green, R. J. (2012). Gay and lesbian family life: Risk, resilience, and rising expectations. In F. Walsh (Ed.), *Normal Family Processes: Growing Diversity and Complexity* (4th ed., pp. 172–195). New York: Guilford Press.

Greenhaus, J. H., & Beutell, N. J. (1985). Sources of conflict between work and family roles. *The Academy of Management Review, 10*(1), 76–88.

Greenstein, T. N. (1996a). Gender ideology and perceptions of the fairness of the division of household labor: Effects on marital quality. *Social Forces, 74*, 1029–1042.

Greenstein, T. N. (1996b). Husbands' participating in domestic labor: Interactive effects of wives' and husbands' gender ideologies. *Journal of Marriage and the Family, 58*, 585–595.

Greenstein, T. N. (2000). Economic dependence, gender, and the division of labor in the home: A replication and extension. *Journal of Marriage and the Family, 62*, 322–335.

Hawkins, A. J., Marshall, C. M., & Allen, S. M. (1998). The orientation toward domestic labor questionnaire: Exploring dual-earner wives' sense of fairness about family work. *Journal of Family Psychology, 12*, 244–258.

Himsel, A. J., & Goldberg, W. A. (2003). Social comparisons and satisfaction with the division of housework: Implications for men's and women's role strain. *Journal of Family Issues, 24*, 843–866.

Horowitz, J. M., Parker, K., Graf, N., & Livingston, G. (2017). *Americans Widely Support Paid Family and Medical Leave, but Differ Over Specific Policies.* Pew Research Center. Retrieved from https://www.pewresearch.org/social-trends/2017/03/23/americ ans-widely-support-paid-family-and-medical-leave-but-differ-over-specific-policies/

Huffman, A. H., Matthews, R. A., & Irving, L. H. (2017). Family fairness and cohesion in marital dyads: mediating processes between work-family conflict and couple psychological distress. *Journal of Occupational and Organizational Psychology, 90*(1), 95–116. http://doi.org/10.1111/joop.12165

Jacobs, J., & Gornick, J. (2001). *Hours of Paid Work in Dual-earner Couples: The US in Cross-national Perspective*. Philadelphia, PA: University of Pennsylvania.

Kluwer, E. S., Heesink, J. A. M., & Van de Vliert, E. (1996). Marital conflict about the division of labor and paid work. *Journal of Marriage and the Family 58*, 958–969.

Kluwer, E. S., Heesink, J. A. M., & Van de Vliert, E. (1997). The marital dynamics of conflict over the division of labor. *Journal of Marriage and the Family 59*, 635–653.

Knudson-Martin, C. (2012). Changing gender norms in families and society: Towards equality amid complexity. In F. Walsh (Ed.), *Normal Family Processes: Growing Diversity and Complexity* (4th ed., pp. 324–346). New York: Guilford Press.

Knudson-Martin, C., & Mahoney, A. R. (2009). Introduction to the special section—Gendered power in cultural contexts: Capturing the lived experience of couples. *Family Process, 48*(1), 5–8. http://dx.doi.org/10.1111/j.1545-5300.2009.01263.x

Korabik, K. (2015). The intersection of gender and work-family guilt. In M. Millis (Ed.), *Gender and the Work-Family Experience*. Cham, Switzerland: Springer.

Kossek, E. E., & Lambert, S. J. (2005). *Work and Life Integration: Organizational, Cultural, and Individual Perspectives*. London: Lawrence Erlbaum Associates.

Kuo, P. X., Volling, B. L., & González, R. (2018). Gender role beliefs, work-family conflict, and father involvement after the birth of a second child. *Psychology of Men & Masculinity. 19*(2), 243.http://doi.org/10.1037/men0000101

Lapierre, L. M., Li, Y., Kwang, H. K., Greenhaus, J. H., Di Renzo, M. S., & Shao, P. (2017). A meta-analysis of the antecedents of work-family enrichment. *Journal of Organizational Behavior, 39*(4), 385–401. http://doi.org/10.1002/job.2234

Lewis, J. (1997). Lone mothers: The British case. In J. Lewis (Ed.), *Lone Mothers in European Welfare Regimes – Shifting Policy Logics*. London: Jessica Kingsley.

Lin, K. J., Llies, R., Pluut, H., & Pan, S. Y. (2017). You are a helpful co-worker, but do you support your spouse? A resource-based work-family model of helping and support provision. *Organizational Behavior and Human Decision Processes, 138*, 45–58. http://doi.org/10.1016/j.obhdp.2016.12.004

Lucas-Thompson, R. G., & Goldberg, W. A. (2015). Gender ideology and work-family plans of the next generation. In M. Mills (Ed.), *Gender and the Work-Family Experience* (pp. 3–19). Cham, Switzerland: Springer.

Major, B. (1987). Gender, justice, and the psychology of entitlement. In P. Shaver & C. Hendrick (Eds), *Sex and Gender* (pp. 124–148). Newbury Park, CA: Sage Publications.

Martínez, M. C., & Paterna, C. (2009). Perspectiva de género aplicada a la conciliación (Gender perspective applied to work-family conciliation). In M. Martinez (Ed.), *Género y Conciliación de la Vida Familiar y Laboral: Un análisis psicosocial* (pp. 17–44). Murcia: Editum-Ediciones de la Universidad de Murcia.

Matias, M., Ferreira, T., Vieira, J., Cadima, J., Leal. T., & Mena Matos, P. (2017). Workplace family support, parental satisfaction, and work-family conflict: individual and crossover effects among dual-earner couples. *Applied Psychology, 66(4)*, 628–652. http://doi.org/10.1111/apps.12103

McGoldrick, M., & Carter, B. (2003). The family life cycle. In F. Walsh (Ed.), *Normal Family Processes: Growing Diversity and Complexity* (3rd ed., pp. 375–398). New York: Guilford Press. http://dx.doi.org/10.4324/9780203428436_chapter_14

McGoldrick, M., & Shibusawa, T. (2012). The family life cycle. In F. Walsh (Ed.), *Normal Family Processes: Growing Diversity and Complexity* (4th ed., pp. 375–398). New York: Guilford Press.

Michel, J. S., & Hargis, B. (2008). Linking mechanisms of work-family conflict and segmentation. *Journal of Vocational Behavior, 73*(3), 509–522. htpp://doi.org/10.1016/j.jvb.2008.09.005

Moen, P., Kaduk, A., Kossek, E. E., Hammer, L., Buxton, O. M., O'Donnell, E., Almeida, D., Fox, K., Tranby, E., Oakes, J. M., & Casper, L. (2015). Is work-family conflict a multilevel stressor linking job conditions to mental health? Evidence from the work, family, and health network. *Research in the Sociology of Work, 26,* 177–217. https://doi.org/10.1108/S0277-283320150000026014

Moore, M. R. (2008). Gendered power relations among women: A study of household decision making in Black, lesbian stepfamilies. *American Sociological Review, 73,* 335–356. http://dx.doi.org/10.1177/000312240807300208

Ollier-Malaterre, A., & Foucreault, A. (2017). Cross-national work-life research: cultural and structural impacts for individuals and organizations. *Journal of Management, 43*(1), 111–136. Htpp://doi.org/10.1177/0149206316655873

Organization for Economic Cooperation and Development (OECD). (2014). *Balancing Paid Work, Unpaid Work and Leisure.* Retrieved from http://www.oecd.org/gender/data/balancingpaidworkunpaidworkandleisure.htm

Papp, L. M., Cummings, E. M., & Goeke-Morey, M. C. (2009). For richer, for poorer: Money as a topic of marital conflict in the home. *Family Relations: An Interdisciplinary Journal of Applied Family Studies, 58*(1), 91–103. http://dx.doi.org/10.1111/j.1741-3729.2008.00537.x

Parker, K., & Funk, C. (2017). *Gender Discrimination Comes in Many Forms for Today's Working Women.* PEW Research. Retrieved from https://www.pewresearch.org/fact-tank/2017/12/14/gender-discrimination-comes-in-many-forms-for-todays-working-women/

Parsons, T., & Bales, R. F. (1955). *Family, Socialization and Interaction Process.* Glencoe, IL: Free Press.

Perry-Jenkins, M., & Folk, K. (1994). Class, couples, and conflict: Effects of the division of labor on assessments of marriage in dual-earner families. *Journal of Marriage and the Family, 56,* 165–180.

Pew Research Center. (2017). *Americans See Men as the Financial Providers, Even as Women's Contributions Grow.* Retrieved from http://www.pewresearch.org/fact-tank/2017/09/20/americans-see-men-as-the-financial-providers-even-as-womens-contributions-grow/

Presser, H. B. (1994). Employment schedules among dual-earner spouses and the division of household labor by gender. *American Sociological Review, 59,* 348–364.

Rogers, S. J., & Amato, P. R. (2000). Have changes in gender relations affected marital quality? *Social Forces, 79,* 731–753.

Sanchez, L. (1994). Gender, labor allocations, and the psychology of entitlement within the home. *Social Forces, 73,* 533–553.

Sanchez, L., & Kane, E. W. (1996). Women's and men's constructions of perceptions of housework fairness. *Journal of Family Issues, 17,* 358–379.

Scanzoni, J. (1982). *Sexual Bargaining: Power Politics in the American Marriage.* Chicago: University of Chicago.

Semega, J., Kollar, M., Shrider, E. A., & Creamer, J. (2020). *US Census Bureau: Income and Poverty in the United States: 2019.* Retrieved from https://www.census.gov/library/publications/2020/demo/p60-270.html

Sprey, J. (1979). Conflict theory and the study of marriage and the family. In W. Burr, R. Hill, F. I. Nye, & I. Reiss (Eds), *Contemporary Theories about the Family, 2* (pp. 130–159). New York: The Free Press.

Steil, J. M. (1997). *Marital Equality: Its Relationship to the Well being of Husbands and Wives.* Thousand Oaks, CA: Sage Series on Close Relationships.

Wayne, J. H., Butts, M. M., Casper, W. J., & Allen, T. (2017). In search of balance: a conceptual and empirical integration of multiple meanings of work-family balance. *Personnel Psychology, 70*(1), 167–210. http://doi.org/10.1111/peps.12132

Westman, M., & Etzion, D. (2005). The crossover of work-family conflict from one spouse to the other. *Journal of Applied Social Psychology, 35*(9), 1936–1957. http://doi.org/10.1111/j.1559-1816.2005.tb02203.x

Wharton, A. S. (2015). 2014 PSA Presidential Address (Un) Changing institutions: work, family and gender in the new economy. *Sociological Perspectives, 58*(1), 7–19. http://doi.org/10.1177/0731121414564471

Wood, W., & Eagly, A. H. (2010). Gender. In S.T. Fiske, D.T. Gilbert, & G. Linzey (Eds), *Handbook of Social Psychology* (pp. 629–667) (5th ed., Vol. 1). Hoboken, NJ: John Wiley & Sons.

11 Awareness of Intersectionality and Self of the Therapist in Training and Supervision

Introduction

Gender is a culturally defined set of perceptions, impacting females' and males' behavior that changes across cultures and time and varies based on power dynamics in every relationship. Understanding the impact of gender on the supervision process and examining how psychotherapists need to be mindful of gender dynamics will be discussed in this chapter. Furthermore, the strong effect of race, racism, and other sociopolitical factors, as well as the person of the therapist throughout the supervision process, will be examined.

Family, school, and media continue to communicate sex-role differences laying out very different sets of appropriate behaviors for boys and girls, generating significantly different psychological environments based on gender. The fact that men as a group often have more economic, political, social, and physical power than most women is the foundation of this discourse. This societal structure contributing to the power differential between men and women creates biases in expectations and behaviors that affect therapy and supervision.

Further, two other factors impact the relationship between men and women and the therapeutic process. Those minimize or exaggerate the significance of the differences between the genders because the within-group differences get ignored. In addition, instead of discussing how gender differences impact women, we need to discuss the fact that bias and discrimination affect both men and women.

Since supervision necessitates managing the process of psychotherapy and gender bias directly impacts the process, three areas are important to consider: (1) the nature of the problems clients discuss in psychotherapy, (2) the psychotherapist's perspective, and (3) the preferences for interventions. Women complain that psychotherapists, perhaps unconsciously, often encourage traditional sex roles and unfair expectations of women. They also complain about the devaluation of female attributes and traits based on sexist theoretical constructs. Thus, supervisors should take the responsibility to help the supervisee consider gender as one of the main factors for case conceptualization, the self of the therapist assessment, and careful consideration for the selection of theoretical approaches.

DOI: 10.4324/9781003088189-12

Gender and Supervision

Since we all live in the same societal contexts, gender issues directly affect the supervisory relationship. According to Bernard and Goodyear (1992), gendered relationships in supervision are directly associated with the structure of the sessions. It is also related to how conflicts are handled, how the feedback gets processed, how satisfying the supervision process is, how comfortable the supervisee feels about disclosing personal struggles, and how the power hierarchy impacts the relationship.

The supervisory relationship is exceptionally important in psychotherapists' personal and professional development. It necessitates a high level of consciousness and recognition of the impact of self and society on the supervisory relationship. Concerning gender, it is vitally important for the supervisors to use the supervisory relationship for educating, confronting, and modeling appropriate therapeutic relationships.

The most crucial aspect is for supervisors to challenge their own preconceptions and biases about gender as a highly sensitive aspect of the supervisory relationship. There must be clear parameters so the supervisor can provide a safe environment for professional and personal development and model proper professional behavior for supervisees. With appropriate training and understanding of the larger social context, supervisors and psychotherapists can work as activists to successfully address inequalities and biases about gender differences. Supervisors can have a long-lasting impact on psychotherapists in training, promoting gender-based fairness and justice by showing authentic awareness of issues both men and women are dealing with in advocating for change in institutions and mental health systems.

Race, Racism, and Supervision

Race is an organizing principle in the everyday lives of so many people in the US and many other countries. The painful social reality of racism impacts psychotherapists and their relationships with their clients (Hardy, 2008). Therefore, it is vitally important to examine the impact of race and racism in supervision. This means that the supervisors are able to hold themselves and the supervisee accountable and discuss the concept of race, racism, and how it impacts the supervisory relationship.

The constructs of race and racism are being more often discussed in the psychotherapy field. It seems like the concept of race is often understood as a socially constructed idea mostly related to skin color. At times religion and culture are also perceived as indicators of racial differences, but it is also connected and confirmed by differences in skin tone. Specifically, how supervisors need to pay attention to these issues and how it impacts the supervisory relationship. This must be perceived as a political issue because the supervisor holds a position of power due to the dominant discourses related to the supervisor being more expert and more experienced (Bobele *et al.*, 1995). The supervisor can use the position of being an expert to either perpetuate the vicious cycle of racism or challenge inequalities between different groups of people. The act of challenging inequalities must be perceived as an ethical act in psychotherapy. The supervisor's responsibility is to initiate conversations about race and racism within the supervisory relationship. Since these discussions are anxiety-provoking and emotionally charged, supervisors must establish a safe context for these relational risks to take place (Mason, 2005). Supervisors must engage their supervisees to self-reflect and process their own racial identity and influence in working with clients and their families. This should be a mutual and consistent process throughout the supervisory relationship.

Gender, Race, and Racism in Psychotherapy

It could be easily claimed that the field of psychotherapy has been another site for the perpetuation of racism, even though the mental health field, as a whole, values and claims to focus on contextual issues in people's lives. The central and powerful systems of racism, sexism, heterosexism, and classism seem to be supported by the theory and practice of psychotherapy. For example, in the field of family therapy, the founders conceptualized the family as white, married, heterosexual, and middle-class, with men being positioned as the head of the household and the woman as the primary custodian of family relationships (McGoldrick & Hardy, 2008). There were no discussions about cultural and racial oppression allowing the perpetuation of the societal systems of domination.

In the 1970s and 1980s, some scholars like Hare-Mustin (1978), James and McIntyre (1983), and Goldner (1988) started writing about the invisibility of discourses about gender in family therapy, even though none discussed the influence of racial issues impacting family relationships. A few years later, scholars like Boyd-Franklin (1989), McGoldrick (1998), Hardy and Laszloffy (2000), and Erskine (2002) started discourses about race and the impact of marginalization on relationships. Nevertheless, the family is still defined in Eurocentric terms by predominantly American and European clinicians who will also teach psychotherapy courses, conduct research, and dominate the discourse about family life.

Thus, psychotherapy must pay close attention to gender and race as the primary organizing principle in everyday life, shaping behaviors, perceptions, and beliefs. Supervisors, then, must discuss the reality of sexism and racism impacting people's lives in every supervision meeting. One of the most significant barriers to avoiding discussing sexism and racism, specifically in a cross-race context, is that it is an emotionally charged subject, given the history of unequal gender and race relationships creating unfair polarizing positions (Erskine, 2002; Hardy, 2008). However, supervisors should have a moral and ethical obligation to challenge gender inequality and racism. The following questions may help supervisors get to know the therapist's understanding of these issues:

1. How do you define your racial identity?
2. How do you define your gender identity?
3. What meanings do you attach to your gender identity?
4. What meanings do you attach to your racial identity?
5. What are the influences of your gender on your intimate relationships?
6. What are the influences of your race on your intimate relationships?
7. How do you think your gender helps or hinders you from connecting with people who define themselves differently than you?
8. How do you think your racial identity helps or hinders you from connecting with people from other races?

This amplified consciousness and compassion ensuing from a process of self-reflection and soul-searching will enable psychotherapists to think about and pay much closer attention to the impact of gender, race, and class on clients presenting problems. It will also help with the supervisors' own responses to the psychotherapists in training. It seems like ethical supervision, which is attuned to the influence of gender, race, and racism, alongside various other forms of oppression influencing people's lives. It is essential to know how supervisors discuss issues related to gender, race, racism, and class, which have implications for the supervisory relationship, which in turn have implications for the therapeutic relationship between supervisees and client families (Arnold, 1993; Burnham & Harris, 2002; Lawless *et al.*, 2001). Issues related to race, culture, and ethnicity should be raised in supervision by the supervisors. If discussions about gender, race, racism, and other contextual factors are not part of the agenda, the supervisees assume that these issues are unimportant, or if they think they are important, they may not discuss them (Garrett *et al.*, 2001; Hird *et al.*, 2001). Further, psychotherapists in training would have way less knowledge and awareness about the influence of gender-based relational patterns, race and racism, and class on their clients' lives. Thus, they will not have the appropriate skill sets to evaluate, develop and provide appropriate and suitable treatment (Hernandez *et al.*, 2009).

It is crucial for the psychotherapists in training to know themselves as cultural beings before exploring cultural influences with their clients (Boyd-Franklin, 2003). Further, according to Hardy and Laszloffy (1997), a cultural genogram can be very helpful to delve into cultural issues advocating for cultural awareness and sensitivity by helping psychotherapists in training to examine their own cultural and racial identities. The cultural genogram can be used in supervision to practice how these issues can be discussed and processed in working with clients. However, the research shows a substantial gap between the supervision literature and the reality of supervisory practice (Lawless *et al.*, 2001). For the most part, it seems like issues related to gender, race, ethnicity, and culture were often only discussed in the context of discussing other clinical problems instead of being raised directly. In a study by Hernandez and his colleagues in 2009, supervisees of color experienced overt racism in their training. The supervisor not only did not provide a safe space for examining these issues, but they also did not address any of the relevant contextual factors either. It is important for the supervision training to be provided based on not just a Eurocentric perspective, which often denies supervisees' and clients' gender and racial identities.

The power differentials that supervisor and supervisee have to be aware of are even more intensified when the supervisor's racial background is white and, unless there is a conscious decision, does not have to address issues related to race and racism (Cook & Helms, 1988; Duan & Roehlke, 2001; Hird *et al.*, 2001). The structure of the supervisory relationship through these discourses leaves the supervisor in the position of power to choose to make these discussions a central part of the supervisory relationship. The systemic supervision with an added postmodern framework must view supervision as a collaborative conversation. The supervisor should utilize a 'not-knowing' stance and participate in mutual meaning-making with the supervisee to motivate supervisees to engage in critical thinking. The supervisor must create a safe space for generating meaningful discourses about gender, race, and racism. They must also help the supervisees develop a better set of skills, have more competence, and have a higher level of expertise (Anderson & Swim, 1995). The supervisor should not leave it to supervisees to bring up issues related to class, gender, race, and marginalization because there are inherently unequal power relations entrenched within the supervisory relationship (Flaskas & Humphreys, 1993; Foucault, 1972). The central discourses concerning gender, race, religion, age, ability, class, culture, ethnicity, education, sexuality, and spirituality, are vital to the supervisees' training. For example, a white, middle-class, Christian, heterosexual, non-disabled, highly educated supervisor should co-construct therapeutic intervention about working with marginalized populations and training a BIPOC (Black, Indigenous, People of Color) female supervisee from different religions and cultures. Similarly, a BIPOC female, middle-class, transgender supervisee must feel comfortable about their own gender and sexual identity and discuss any issues related to their intersectionality and therapeutic skills set in supervision so they can work with other marginalized groups.

Thus, discussing gender, race, class, disabilities, religion, and other issues should always be the first step in supervisory discourses. As a female, Muslim, middle-class, heterosexual supervisor, I have been mainly supervising white male and female supervisees. However, I have also supervised many BIPOC and sexual minority supervisees. In every supervision encounter, I would assume that while my gender and religion may create complex power dynamics, my extensive supervisory experience and academic positions would allow me to have a higher level of power than my supervisees. Thus, when we consult about cases, we always map out how the supervisee's intersectionality impacts the way they view the issue and understand the intersectionality of their clients' positions. My supervisory position grants me the power to have much more significant influence in discourses, intensified by my experience. However, given that my own intersectional identities are complex, I discuss my own developmental process and engage my supervisees to discuss these issues. I perceive power dynamics in both supervisory and therapeutic relationships as interrelated and central to ethical supervision. Therefore, I provide a context where discourses about gender, religion, sexual orientation, race, and racism are part of every discussion.

Byng-Hall (1995) stated that supervisors must see themselves as attachment figures needing to create a safe base for their supervisees to feel protected and supported to explore and learn therapeutic skills. They must process any issues related to self that may come up and be encouraged to explore different ways clients may need their support. Then, this isomorphic process gives the supervisees the security to create a safe context for working with their clients and be a source of secure attachment for them. It may be helpful to discuss the supervisee's family of origin influences in supervision sessions, so the supervisees can talk about their intersectional identities and their relationships with clients. For example, during the initial supervision sessions, I often talk about how my father believed that gender was a social construct and men and women should be equally treated based on their skills and talents. I discuss how his perspectives shaped my views about my social positions. I also talk about being raised in an upper-class family but being continuously challenged to understand the privilege of having access to resources without judging the working class and how these values shaped my identity of consistently advocating for those with less privilege.

On the other hand, I discuss how being a Muslim woman from Iran has shaped my professional identity and how people see me as an oppressed woman regardless of my academic and professional positions, which create a double consciousness for me needing to continuously be aware of my sense of self and how others perceive me. The supervisors' responsibility is to make sure supervisees are aware and accountable for their cultural, racial, class, spiritual, and many other identities and know the impact of their intersectionality on their therapeutic work with clients. This often models a self-introspective process for the supervision group to examine their social locations concerning gender, race, ethnicity, culture, religion, and class, among many others.

Self of the Therapist

There is strong research indicating that it is the psychotherapist and not the psychotherapy model that impacts the outcome of the therapeutic process (Blow *et al.*, 2007). There has also been a clear emphasis on training psychotherapists to be conscious in using their personal selves in the therapy process (Aponte, 1994; Aponte & Winter, 2000; Aponte & Kissil, 2012: D'Aniello & Fife, 2020; Satir, 2000; Simon, 2006, 2012; Wampold & Imel, 2015; Niño *et al.*, 2015). Harry Aponte (2017) has developed a model for training therapists called the Person-of-the-Therapist Training model to expand psychotherapists' success irrespective of therapy models. In his model, self-awareness is the hallmark of training in the context of the therapeutic process.

Person-of-the-therapist clinical supervision focuses on the professional and personal elements of the therapeutic process. Theoretically, psychotherapists adopt a therapy model based on a philosophical perspective with some guidelines for assessment and interventions to help clients change. However, the psychotherapists must use themselves to build trust with clients and develop compassion in order to carry out their interventions. Thus, all forms of psychotherapy must rely on a strong connection between professional techniques and personal connections.

From the beginning of the formation of talk therapy by Freud (1964), since the psychoanalyst and the patient had to rely on their relationships, Freud believed understanding countertransference could be very helpful. Bowen (1972), trained in psychoanalysis and a founder of a family therapy model, also spoke about the need for training therapists to encounter clients. Bowen's personal journey to differentiate himself from his family became a hallmark of his model and a great training source for therapists to differentiate themselves from their families of origin. Virginia Satir (2000) also advocated for therapists to work on their issues "with his or her own family" (p. 21), achieving a sense of "integrated self" (p. 24). Today, most supervision training emphasizes examining family roles and unsettled relational tensions affecting therapy and supervision (Todd & Storm, 1997). According to Rober (1999), there are the therapist's outer and therapeutic conversations, with the inner dialogue being between the person-of-the-therapist and the professional self of the therapist. Rober believed that therapeutic gridlocks happen when psychotherapists have not dealt with the inner blocks within their own sense of selves. Overall, the person-of-the-therapist model can be used with any therapeutic model, focusing on the psychotherapists' conscious and deliberate use of self in the therapy room. The supervisory model is also based on the same 'self of the therapist model.'

Self of the Supervisor

Culturally diverse societies cannot deal with only one set of norms applied to all members in any therapeutic setting since conforming to societal standards for healthy functioning is no longer a viable option. People choose different lifestyles. They decide on various ways to have children and when and how they may choose to die. They define their own sexual identities, and more people fight for having choices and don't value strict commitments and obligations. In individualistically oriented nations like the US, personal freedom prioritizes collective decision-making, and equality is more valued.

Thus, the traditional Eurocentric therapeutic interventions based on intact white middle-class Christian families can no longer be the only way we understand diverse family functioning. We have witnessed new development in social justice perspectives and psychotherapists working with specific populations such as the LGBTQT community. These perspectives impact the underlying philosophy for mental health practices. Therefore, we must strive to train psychotherapists that are not value-neutral and take political and social actions into account as part of their intervention approaches. Psychotherapy has become less hierarchical and more collaborative. Clients are demanding to know more about the therapists' values, and self-disclosure is appreciated and welcomed. The therapy models are more outcome-based and action-oriented, psychotherapists are more active, their interventions are value-based, and they are more emotionally and personally invested in the therapy process. Hence, it makes great sense for psychotherapists to take more responsibility for conducting therapy. Psychotherapists' self-awareness must be central to their mastery of therapeutic interventions and professional processes. Therefore, training and supervision based on the emotional, cultural, and spiritual use of self are needed.

Person-of-the-Therapist Supervision Model

The main goal of supervision is to assist psychotherapists in providing more effective therapy with their clients. Supervision primarily focuses on the detail of the case, linking client issues with developmental and relational sources, and utilizing approaches to achieve therapy's objectives. The supervisees' personal gain is secondary to the supervisory process. Still, central to this clinical effort is the ongoing and intentional use of self in the therapeutic process from evaluation to intervention. The supervisor must support the therapist's use of self and the practical and professional aspects of the therapeutic process. The intensity of the issues the supervisors examine in supervision depends on the demands of the case and the supervisees' skills in dealing with their therapist's role. Psychotherapists interested in their own growth must utilize these types of supervision more than those who see the therapeutic process as using a set of techniques and assessment tools. Further, supervisors helping supervisees with the intersectionality of their identities are better positioned to help supervisees succeed in their therapeutic work with clients.

Given that the person-of-the-therapist's work is not linked to any therapy model, it can be used with all therapy schools. It is about holding supervisees accountable for their personal development and being conscious of the sense of self utilized in every aspect of therapy. The most important part of the self-of-the-therapist's work is its centrality in the context of a relationship with a client for assessment and intervention. Therapists' cultural, ethical, relational, and spiritual values are considered as the primary contexts for therapists' decision-making process and choices of interventions. Supervisors must help therapists take responsibility for their beliefs and worldviews and see them as the foundation of their therapeutic work with clients.

Person-of-the-Therapist Supervision Tool

Aponte and Winter (2000) developed an important supervision instrument using self-of-the-therapist's perspective. The instrument focuses on the case's practical and clinical challenges and uses the therapist's personal information concerning the client's issues. Then, the clients' problems are discussed and linked to the therapist's personal information to see how to use the self of the therapist in the diagnostic and interventional aspects of therapy. The fundamental idea "concentrates primarily on the bridge between the actual conduct of treatment and the therapist's personal life" (Aponte & Winter, 2000: 145). The instrument has an instruction sheet and evaluation sheet, including the Person-of-the-Therapist supervisory form. The form must be completed for each case and utilized for every supervisory session. The critical step is for therapists to foresee how they can use themselves in therapy, from formulating a hypothesis to the therapeutic goals and then executing the therapeutic strategy and technical interventions.

Person-of-the-Therapist Supervision Instrument (Adopted by permission from Harry J. Aponte and J. Carol Carlsen)

1. Provide identifying information about the client:

   _____

2. Attach the client's genogram:

   _____

3. State the agreed-upon issue the client is seeking help for in therapy, and note anything in it that carries personal meaning for you:

   _____

4. Describe your personal reactions to your clients and theirs to you:

   _____

5. Address whatever cultural or spiritual values may be coloring how you view the issues they are presenting as distinct from your client's perspectives:

   _____

6. State the aspect of the issue you aim to deal with in today's supervisory session, and highlight anything in it that carries personal meaning for you:

   _____

7. Explicate your hypotheses about the roots and dynamics of the client's issue:

_____

8. Explain your therapeutic strategy with the case, and in particular with the aspects of the case you are to discuss in today's supervision:

_____

9. Detail how you are implementing your strategy's technical interventions:

_____

10. Detail how you use yourself in conjunction with your interventions:

_____

11. Identify your personal challenges working with this client around the focal issue:

_____

12. Discuss your plan for meeting your personal challenges in this case:

_____

General Instruction for Using Person-of-the-Therapist Supervision

General

- The supervisor and supervisees can use any therapeutic model if they choose to use this instrument.
- Personal and professional boundaries are critical. Thus, the personal question should directly relate to the case, and no other personal information should be elicited.
- The main objective is to incorporate the technical and personal mechanisms of the therapeutic process. The supervisor must ensure that the clinical and personal observations are intertwined and interconnected, and there are always clear boundaries between the two.

Specific

- #1: Provide only factual information, and not the reason clients are seeking therapy.
- #2: The genogram should not be very detailed, and the discussion should be more about the link between what aspects of the family genogram have personal significance for the supervisee.
- #3: Provide a very concise, specific synopsis about the clients' issues with a comment about personal relevance for the therapist.
- #4: Describe the relationship between client and therapist and its possible influence on the therapeutic relationship.
- #5: Discuss therapist's cultural values, spirituality, personal standards, what seems functional and dysfunctional based on both the client and the therapist's values, including the suitability of resolutions and goals.
- #6: Discuss any issues that the client is bringing up that have a personal connection.
- #7: Discuss the hypotheses and the reason for the suggested solutions.
- #8: Discuss the use of many techniques and the therapeutic models.
- #9: Discuss the technical process and the nature of the therapeutic relationship.
- #10 Describe the use of the self-of-the-therapist in technical interventions and the therapeutic relationships.
- #11: It is imperative to discuss personal challenges related to personal or technical aspects of the treatment and interventions.
- #12: Discuss the types of solutions and the kind of help the therapist needs for these personal challenges.

Conclusion

Gender, culture, race, class, and many other identifying markers organize our own lives and our interactions with our clients in the therapy room in intense and meaningful ways. These identifying markers continue to be essential aspects of our clients' lives, impacting their everyday experiences (Christiansen *et al.*, 2009). Thus, it is utterly important to make these discourses part of the systemic supervision and expect supervisors to be responsible for creating a safe context due to their power over the supervisee. This makes sense ethically, but it has to start with the supervisor creating a safe context for supervisees to feel comfortable taking relational risks and examining these systemic issues impacting their clients' lives daily.

The Person-of-the-Therapist Supervision Instrument can help supervisees examine their skills in making effective use of themselves in the therapy room. This instrument can be utilized to provide quality feedback to therapists about their awareness of their conscious self in offering therapy and developing specific competencies to use self for the therapeutic process. It also demands a focus on the person of the supervisor. Each supervision session then can end with evaluating the supervision process and what was or was not helpful to the therapist. Further, the essential aspect of supervision is the parallel process between the therapist's own sense of growth and their work with clients. This process also necessitates the supervisors examining their own use of self and its impact on the supervisory process. It is important to note that the extensive use of self in therapy is a very personal undertaking embedded in the therapeutic process. Therefore, supervisors need to be responsive, insightful, and wise in their attempt to help the supervisee with their soul searching to get to know themselves to understand their clients' pain, connect with them fully, and enable them to change. The training is also necessary for supervisors to develop proficiency in using their own developed self to facilitate a change process for their supervisees. This will help therapists continuously take the risk of examining their own abilities and vulnerabilities to provide the best possible care for their clients.

These discussions must be part of the supervision process to maintain an ethical supervisory and therapeutic practice. Examining one's gendered identity, class, religion, sexual orientation, and many other intersections of our identities helps us develop better skills in providing ethically and morally appropriate psychotherapy. One can argue that this is the only way to bring about change at the relationship level and then at the societal level. Anything less cannot serve our clients well and is simply not good enough for a field that must make every effort to help clients with issues related to social justice and the eradication of inequality.

References

Anderson, H., & Swim, S. (1995). Supervision as collaborative conversation: connecting the voices of supervisor and supervisee. *Journal of Systemic Therapies, 14,* 1–13.
Aponte, H. J. (1994). *Bread & Spirit: Therapy with the New Poor.* New York: Norton.
Aponte, H. J. (2017). The philosophy of the person-of-the-therapist training model: The underlying premises. *Seminare; Learned Investigations, 38*(4), 57–67. https:// doi. org/ 10. 21852/ sem. 2017,4. 05
Aponte, H., & Carlsen, J. (2009). An Instrument for Person-of-the-Therapist Supervision. *Journal of Marital and Family Therapy, 35,* 395–405. http://doi.org/ 10.1111/j.1752-0606.2009.00127.x
Aponte, H. J., & Kissil, K. (2012). "If I can grapple with this, I can truly be of use in the therapy room": Using the therapist's own emotional struggles to facilitate effective therapy. *Journal of Marital & Family Therapy, 40*(2), 152–164. https:// doi. org/ 10.1111/ jmft. 12011
Aponte, H. J., & Winter, J. E. (2000). The person and practice of the therapist: Treatment and training. In M. Baldwin (Ed.), *The Use of Self in Therapy* (2nd ed., pp. 127–166). New York: Haworth.
Arnold, M. S. (1993). Ethnicity and training marital and family therapists. *Counselor Education and Supervision, 33,* 139–147.

Bernard, J. M. & Goodyear, R. K. (1992). *Fundamentals of Clinical Supervision*. Boston, MA: Allyn and Bacon.

Blow, A. J., Sprenkle, D. H., & Davis, S. D. (2007). Is who delivers the treatment more important than the treatment itself? The role of the therapist in common factors. *Journal of Marital and Family Therapy, 33*(3), 298–317. https:// doi. org/ 10. 1111/ j.1752- 0606. 2007. 00029.x

Bobele, M., Gardner, G., & Biever, J. (1995). Supervision as social construction. *Journal of Systemic Therapies, 14,* 4–25.

Boyd-Franklin, N. (1989). *Black Families in Therapy*. New York: Guilford Press.

Boyd-Franklin, N. (2003). *Black Families in Therapy: Understanding the African American Experience*. New York: Guilford.

Bowen, M. (1972). Toward a differentiation of a self in one's family. In James L. Framo (Ed.), *Family Interaction* (pp. 111–173). New York: Springer.

Burnham, J., & Harris, Q. (2002). Cultural issues in supervision. In D. Campbell & B. Mason (Eds), *Perspectives on Supervision* (pp. 21–41). London: Karnac.

Byng-Hall, J. (1995). *Rewriting Family Scripts: Improvisation and Systems Change*. New York: Guilford Press.

Christiansen, A. T., Thomas, V., Kafescioglu, N., Karakurt, G., Lowe, W., Smith, W., & Wittenborn, A. (2009). Multicultural supervision: lessons learned about an ongoing struggle. *Journal of Marital and Family Therapy, 35*(1), 1–11.

Cook, D. A., & Helms, J. E. (1988). Visible racial/ethnic group supervisees' satisfaction with cross-cultural supervision as predicted by relationship characteristics. *Journal of Counseling Psychology, 35,* 268–274.

D'Aniello, C., & Fife, S. T. (2020). A 20-year review of common factors research in marriage and family therapy: A mixed methods content analysis. *Journal of Marital and Family Therapy, 46*(4), 701–718.

Duan, C., & Roehlke, H. (2001). A descriptive "snapshot" of cross-racial supervision in university counseling center internships. *Journal of Multicultural Counseling and Development, 29,* 131–146.

Erskine, R. (2002). Exposing racism, exploring race. *Journal of Family Therapy, 24,* 282–297.

Flaskas, C., & Humphreys, C. (1993). Theorizing about power: intersecting the ideas of Foucault with the "problem" of power in family therapy. *Family Process, 32,* 35–47.

Foucault, M. (1972). *The Archaeology of Knowledge and the Discourse on Language*. (Trans. A. Sheridan). New York: Pantheon Books.

Freud, S. (1964). Analysis terminable and interminable. In J. Strachey (Ed. & Trans.), *The Standard Edition of the Complete Psychological Works of Sigmund Freud* (Vol. 22, p. 249). London: Hogarth Press. (Original work published 1937)

Garrett, M. T., Borders, L. D., Crutchfield, L. B., Torres-Rivera, E., Brotherton, D., & Curtis, R. (2001). Multicultural supervision: a paradigm of cultural responsiveness for supervisors. *Journal of Multicultural Counseling and Development, 29,* 147–158.

Goldner, V. (1988). Generation and gender: normative and covert hierarchies. *Family Process, 27,* 17–31.

Hardy, K. V. (2008). Race, reality and relationships: implications for the re-visioning of family therapy. In M. McGoldrick & K. V. Hardy (Eds.), *Re-Visioning Family Therapy* (2nd ed., pp.76–84). New York: Guilford Press.

Hardy, K. V., & Laszloffy, T. A. (1997). The cultural genogram: an application. In T. Todd & C. Storm (Eds), *The Complete Systemic Supervisor Resource Guide* (pp. 34–39). Boston: Allyn & Bacon.

Hardy, K. V., & Laszloffy, T. A. (2000). Uncommon strategies for a common problem: addressing racism in family therapy. *Family Process*, *39*, 35–50.

Hare-Mustin, R. (1978). A feminist approach to family therapy. *Family Process*, *17*, 181–194.

Hernandez, P., Taylor, B. A., & McDowell, T. (2009). Listening to ethnic minority AAMFT-approved supervisors: reflections on their experiences as supervisees. *Journal of Systemic Therapies*, *28*, 88–100.

Hird, J., Cavalieri, C., Dulko, J., Felice, A., & Ho, T. (2001). Visions and realities: supervisee perspectives of multicultural supervision. *Journal of Multicultural Counseling and Development*, *29*, 114–130.

James, K., & McIntyre, D. (1983). The reproduction of families: the social role of family therapy? *Journal of Marital and Family Therapy*, *9*, 119–129.

Lawless, J. J., Gale, J. E., & Bacigalupe, G. (2001). The discourse of race and culture in family therapy supervision: a conversational analysis. *Contemporary Family Therapy*, *23*, 181–197.

McGoldrick, M. (Ed.) (1998). *Re-visioning Family Therapy*. New York: Guilford Press.

McGoldrick, M., & Hardy, K. V. (2008). Introduction: re-visioning family therapy from a multicultural perspective. In M. McGoldrick & K.V. Hardy (Eds.), *Re-visioning Family Therapy* (2nd ed., pp. 3–19). New York: Guilford Press.

Mason, B. (2005). Relational risk-taking and the training of supervisors. *Journal of Family Therapy*, *27*, 298–301.

Niño, A., Kissil, K., & Apolinar Claudio, F. L. (2015). Perceived professional gains of master's level students following a person of the therapist training program: A retrospective content analysis. *Journal of Marital and Family Therapy*, *41*(2), 163–176. https://doi. org/ 10. 1111/ jmft. 12051

Rober, P. (1999). The therapist's inner conversation in family therapy practice: Some ideas about the self of the therapist, therapeutic impasse, and the process of reflection. *Family Process*, *38*, 209–228.

Satir, V. (2000). The therapist story. In M. Baldwin (Ed.), *The Use of Self in Therapy* (2nd ed., pp. 17–27). New York: Haworth.

Simon, G. M. (2006). The heart of the matter: a proposal for placing the self of the therapist at the center of family therapy research and training. *Family Process*, *45*, 331–344.

Simon, G. M. (2012). The role of the therapist: What effective therapists do. *Journal of Marital and Family Therapy*, *38*(1), 8–12. https:// doi. org/ 10. 1111/j. 1752- 0606. 2009. 00136.x

Todd, T. C., & Storm, C. L. (1997). *The Complete Systemic Supervisor*. Boston, MA: Allyn & Bacon.

Wampold, B. E., & Imel, Z. E. (2015). *The Great Psychotherapy Debate: The Evidence for What Makes Psychotherapy Work*. Abingdon: Routledge.

12 Conclusion

Introduction

Social justice and mental health seem to be located far away from each other. Social justice is defined as justice in distributing wealth, opportunities, and privileges in a society. On the other hand, mental health supposedly resides inside an individual. However, those who suffer from many disadvantages in society also suffer from more significant mental health issues. For example, Sheppard (2002) examines the meaningful relationships between gender and depression and race and schizophrenia, indicating severe psychological consequences for people experiencing social injustices.

Throughout this book, we have discussed gender in terms of societal expectations and perceptions of how we should think and act as women and men. There is an unjust treatment of those who don't see themselves in this binary continuum and don't define themselves based on a binary and static definition of sex. Gender equality and justice become a reality when there is an absence of discrimination based on a person's sex in opportunities, the distribution of resources, and access to services for all people regardless of sex and sexual orientation. It is important to note that there is no denying gender differences based on biomedical issues such as genetic, hormonal, anatomical, and physiological. There are psychosocial differences such as personality, coping, symptom manifestation, and epidemiological differences related to the population-based risk factors. More global differences are based on cultural, social, financial, and political practices that eventually generate health disparity for women and men (Cislaghi, et al., 2020; Kawachi et al., 1999).

Nevertheless, health inequity is seldom based on biology alone. Societal factors, including gender, influence and intensify biological vulnerabilities. For example, psychosocial risks accrue throughout life and significantly enhance the chances of inadequate mental health and early death (World Health Organization, 2001). Mental health issues significantly contribute to the global problem of disease and disability. Mental and behavioral disorders contribute to disability for men and women. Moreover, large disparities in population coverage rates exist between high- and low-income countries. According to the World Health Organization (WHO), by 2011 only 60 percent of its member

DOI: 10.4324/9781003088189-13

countries had mental health policies, while 71 percent created specific mental health procedures and only 59 percent had specific regulations about mental health related issues (World Health Organization, 2011).

Over the years, general medical practitioners have seen more women receive services for mental disorders in primary care settings than men, but this does not mean that they receive adequate mental health services. Thus, clinicians need help from the medical professionals, especially from epidemiologists and epidemiologically based research, to understand for what gender and under what circumstance there are higher risks of experiencing psychological distress and mental illness ((World Health Organization, 2001).

Gender and Mental Health

The main goal of this book is to examine gender, power, and social justice, focusing on honoring gender differences in providing psychotherapy. Overall, based on the strong interconnection between gender and health, even though the distinction between biological and social factors is essential, there is also a strong connection between gender inequality and health outcomes. A gender-sensitive approach to mental health should combine proper responses from the mental healthcare system and public policy. Regardless of socioeconomic status, gender differences impact men and women differently. Research shows that never married, separated, and divorced men's rates of admission to mental health services are higher than those of women with the same marital status categories. On the other hand, married women have higher admission rates than married men.

Furthermore, gender is not a separate phenomenon acting in isolation. It directly interacts with other social indicators like class and race, revealing that working-class and marginalized BIPOC individuals suffer from a higher incidence of unrecognized mental health problems. A systemic gender, class, and race analysis expands our awareness and perceptions of the epidemiology of mental health problems, helps us with better policymaking and proper treatment for marginalized groups, and enhances public health participation (Vlassoff & Garcia Moreno, 2002). Overlooking gender and other intersectional differences and not recognizing gender and race bias can have severe outcomes. Women are more likely to be diagnosed with depression than men, even with comparable scores on standardized measures of depression, and even when they present identical symptoms. Gender impacts the way we perceive and stigmatize emotional problems in women and chemical dependency, especially alcoholism, in men. There is a higher prevalence of the diagnosis of schizophrenia for black men and conduct disorder for black adolescent boys, which reveals a huge stumbling block for the proper identification and treatment of psychological disorders (World Health Organization, 2006). Women's mental health impacts their work productivity and the mental health of their children and elderly parents. Additionally, adolescent girls' mental health disorders such as mood, anxiety, and eating disorders can have a long-lasting effect on their functioning. The same can be true for alcoholism and the externalizing manifestation of mental health issues impacting adolescent boys.

Gender and Health Seeking

Observing health through a gender lens requires actions to enhance women's access, affordability, and suitability of health services. It seems clear that with the gender disparities in health, the medical services without proper mental health services are clearly inadequate (Ahmed *et al.*, 2000; Kumari, 2020). Women's health services are often more related to reproductive health, disregarding women's needs outside the reproductive ages. Poor women also have less access to healthcare than men from the same social group, even in a developed country like the United States (Borchelt, 2022; Krieger & Zierler, 1995). In other countries, women suffer from a lack of confidentiality and having access to information about alternative options and available services (Vlassoff, 1994). Other issues are related to either misdiagnosis or prescribing the wrong medication (Keers *et al.*, 2018; Malterud & Okkes, 1998; World Health Organization, 1998). Moreover, the social acceptability of sick roles on the one hand and the emotional and cognitive capabilities of women for endurance, on the other hand, make health-seeking behavior more complicated (Stangl *et al.*, 2019; Papanek, 1988). According to Amin and Bentley (2002), gender inequalities for women reveal themselves in fertility, marriage, work standards, violence in marital relationships, and inadequate psychological health, forcing women to accept higher tolerances for suffering and not seeking treatment for their symptoms.

Gender and Mental Health Disorder

According to the findings of a study by Astbury (2006), gender differences in mental disorders go beyond the illness's rates, onset, or course. They include many factors impacting susceptibility, diagnosis, treatment, and adjustment to mental disorders. For example, there are apparent gender differences in the prevalence of mental disorders in different age groups. For example, adolescent boys are three times more likely to be diagnosed with conduct disorder (Patel *et al.*, 2018; Scott, 1988), while adolescent girls have a higher prevalence of depression eating disorders. On the other hand, girls engage more in suicidal ideation and suicide attempts than boys, while boys are more susceptible to more risky behaviors and commit suicide more frequently (Hawton *et al.*, 2002; Parker & Roy, 2001). During adulthood, women have a higher frequency of being diagnosed with affective disorders and non-affective psychosis, and men have higher ratios of substance use disorders and antisocial personality disorder (Linzer *et al.*, 1996). Men and women act in response to stress differently, with men developing antisocial behavior and alcohol abuse of being socialized to express anger and acting out behavior. In contrast, women express dysphoria in response to stress.

Men in Therapy

The culturally based ideologies we all use to provide therapy to men create a context for possibly mistreating men. The therapy literature in Britain and North America does not offer many more specific tools and strategies for working with men than for women. Much of the therapeutic literature centering on men's issues is based on the psychoanalytic tradition (Erickson, 1993, 1998; Frosh, 1994). The family therapy literature that has tried to address therapy with men (Lazur, 1998; Bograd, 1991a; Dienhart & Avis, 1990; Dienhart & Dollahite, 1997; Erickson, 1993; Meth & Pasick, 1990) frequently treated men as generic and has not focused on different race or ethnicity, class, or sexual orientation. Specifically, this literature does not pay attention to working with men in family therapy, which requires a different set of skills based on the gender of the therapist and the collection of assumptions about gender patterns in families. The counseling psychology literature in the US suggests that female psychotherapists focus more on issues challenging the traditional male gender roles. There is also literature about men's struggle to stay away from feminine traits, while also having the desire to attach to the feminine side, and the acknowledgment of male defensiveness needing continual patience by the female therapist (Birk, 1981; Bograd, 1991b; Carlson, 1981; Erickson, 1993; Slive, 1986).

The specific issues for male therapists are often related to power, intimacy, and pain (Scher, 1981). Male therapists have a remarkable opportunity to act as powerful role models, exhibiting behaviors, values, and beliefs that can challenge male gender stereotypes. The male therapist can also support the male client deal with his own socialized constraints to his true humanity (Morgan, 1981; O'Neil, 1981; Reimers & Dimmock, 1990; Scher, 1981). Dienhart (2001) states that it may be possible for men to experience greater satisfaction and be willing to do more self-reflection with female psychotherapists. This clinical literature signifies that men's socialization creates difficulties for therapists working on the process of change. Moreover, due to the power differences between white men and men of color, there are even more difficulties with using gender, power, and social justice perspectives in working with men.

Conclusion

Successful approaches to reducing mental health risk factors must be gender-sensitive because women's status and life opportunities remain low worldwide, contributing to higher risks for mental health problems. Cross-culturally, women struggle with self-worth, competency, self-sufficiency, adequate income, and fair access to physical, sexual, and psychological well-being and security, which are fundamental for mental health, and are routinely denied. The widespread violation of women's rights, including controlling their reproductive rights, impacts them directly, causing poor mental health. Hence, an inter-disciplinary action to create policies to protect and promote women's self-sufficiency and independence to lower women's mental health symptoms is necessary. There is a great need for a gender-based data collection and analysis systems to monitor women's and men's health issues more appropriately. There has to be an integration of gender-relevant markers in the existing national health information systems in all nations to monitor gender sensitivity in the health system.

There are differences beyond the prevalence rates of mental disorders and other diseases due to men and women's roles and duties, societal positions, and access to and use of health resources. Primary care providers and mental health professionals need to be sensitive to gender as well as other intersectional identities. Linking gender and cultural sensitivity to training and performance assessments ensures better translation to practice. The entire health system must pay more attention to identifying indicators to increase coping skills, lower stress, and design intervention programs at the community and national levels. It is critical to examine and improve community services and engage non-governmental organizations to protect and foster men's, women's, and marginalized groups' interdependence, self-reliance, and mental health.

This book deliberately attempted to focus on the intersection of gender, power, and social justice within the global context, aiming to create a balanced perspective about the relational dynamics of men and women in heterosexual and homosexual relationships utilizing the healing power of psychotherapy. It approached issues from the biological, sociological, contextual, and ecological perspectives and combined these insights with a clinical approach providing readers with the tools and skills necessary to provide psychotherapy.

Further, it delved into topics such as nature, nurture, masculinity, women's issues, the impact of Western colonization, politics, religion, war, violence, work, as well as race and class and their impact on our everyday gendered interactions. The main goal was to promote justice in our gendered relationships and highlight how we can anti-pathologize symptoms and deal with the implications of socio-political, cultural, and relational issues in our therapeutic practice. The ultimate goal is to be emotionally grounded, relationally congruent, and sociopolitically conscious psychotherapists.

References

Ahmed, S. M., Adams, A. M., Chowdhury, M., & Bhuiya, A. (2000). Gender, socio-economic development and health-seeking behavior in Bangladesh. *Social Science & Medicine, 51*(3), 361–371.

Amin, A., & Bentley, M. E. (2002). The influence of gender on rural women's illness experiences and health-seeking strategies for gynecological symptoms. *Journal of Health Management, 4*(2), 229–249.

Astbury, J. (2006). *Gender and Mental Health.* Paper presented under the Global Health Equity Initiative (GHEI) project on "Gender and Health Equity" based at the Harvard Center for Population and Development Studies. Retrieved from www.grhf.harvard.edu/HUpapers/gender/astbury.pdf.

Birk, J. M. (1981). Relevance and alliance: cornerstones in training counselors of men. *The Personal and Guidance Journal, 60*(4), 259–262.

Bograd, M. (Ed.). (1991a). *Feminist Approaches for Men in Family Therapy*. New York: The Hawthorn Press.

Bograd, M. (1991b). Female therapist/male client: considerations about systems. In M. Bograd (Ed.), *Feminist Approaches for Men in Family Therapy* (pp. 123–152). New York: The Hawthorn Press.

Borchelt, G. (2022). The impact poverty has on women's health. *Human Rights Magazine, 43* (3). https://www.americanbar.org/groups/crsj/publications/human_rights_magazine_home/the-state-of-healthcare-in-the-united-states/poverty-on-womens-health/

Carlson, N. (1981). Male client – female therapist. *Personal and Guidance Journal, 60*(4), 228–231.

Cislaghi, B., Weber, A. M., Gupta, G. R., & Darmstadt, G. L. (2020). Gender equality and global health: intersecting political challenges. *Journal of Global Health, 10*(1), 010701. https://doi.org/10.7189/jogh.10.010701

Dienhart, A. (2001). Engaging men in family therapy: does the gender of the therapist make a difference? *Journal of Family Therapy, 23*(1), 21–45.

Dienhart, A., & Avis, J. M. (1990). Men in therapy: exploring feminist-informed alternatives. *Journal of Feminist Family Therapy, 2*, 25–50.

Dienhart, A., & Dollahite, D. C. (1997). A generative narrative approach to clinical work with fathers. In A. J. Hawkins & D. C. Dollahite (Eds), *Generative Fathering: Beyond Deficit Perspectives* (pp. 183–199). Thousand Oaks, CA: Sage.

Erickson, B. (1998). Ethical considerations when feminist family therapists treatment. *Journal of Feminist Family Therapy, 7*(2), 1–19.

Erickson, B. (1993) *Helping Men Change: The Role of the Female Therapist*. Newbury Park, CA: Sage.

Frosh, S. (1994). *Sexual Difference: Masculinity and Psychoanalysis*. New York: Routledge.

Hawton, K., Rodham, K., Evans, E., & Weatherall, R. (2002). Deliberate self-harm in adolescents: self-report survey in schools in England. *BMJ, 325*(7374), 1207–1211.

Kawachi, I., Kennedy, B. P., Gupta, V., & Prothrow-Sith, D. (1999). Women's status and the health of women and men: a view from the States. *Social Science & Medicine, 48*(1), 21–32.

Keers, R. N., Plácido, M., Bennett, K., Clayton, K., Brown, P., *et al.* (2018) What causes medication administration errors in a mental health hospital? A qualitative study with nursing staff. PLOS ONE 13(10): e0206233. https://doi.org/10.1371/journal.pone.0206233

Krieger, N., & Zierler, S. (1995). Accounting for the health of women. *Current Issues Public Health, 11*, 251–256.

Kumari, P. (2020). Study of gender differences in mental health. *International Journal of Physiology, Nutrition and Physical Education, 5*(2): 226–228

Lazur, R. F. (1998). Men in the family: A family system's approach to treating men. In W. S. Pollack & R. F. Levant (Eds.), *New Psychotherapy for Men* (pp. 127–144). Hoboken, NJ: John Wiley & Sons.

Linzer, M., Spitzer, R., Kroenke, K., Williams, J. B., Hahn, S., Brody, D., & DeGruy, F. (1996). Gender, quality of life, and mental disorders in primary care: results from the PRIME-MD 1000 study. *The American Journal of Medicine, 101*(5), 526–533.

Malterud, K., & Okkes, I. (1998). Gender differences in general practice consultations: methodological challenges in epidemiological research. *Family Practice, 15*(5), 404–410.

Meth, R., & Pasick, R. (1990). *Men in Therapy: The Challenge of Change*. New York: Guilford Press.

Morgan, R. M. (1981). Counselling the uncoupling male. *Personal and Guidance Journal, 60*(4), 237–240.

O'Neil, J. M. (1981). Patterns of gender role conflict and strain: sexism and fear of femininity in men's lives. *Personal and Guidance Journal, 60*(4), 203–209.

Papanek, H. (1988). To each less than she needs, from each more than she can do: allocations, entitlements and value. In I. Tinker (Ed.), *Persistent Inequalities: Women and World Development*. Oxford: Oxford University Press.

Parker, G., & Roy, K. (2001). Adolescent depression: a review. *Australian & New Zealand Journal of Psychiatry, 35*(5), 572–580.

Patel, R. S., Amaravadi, N., Bhullar, H., Lekireddy, J., & Win, H. (2018). Understanding the demographic predictors and associated comorbidities in children hospitalized with conduct disorder. *Behavioral Sciences (Basel, Switzerland), 8*(9), 80. https://doi.org/ 10.3390/bs8090080

Prata, N. (2009). Making family planning accessible in resource-poor settings. *Philosophical Transactions of the Royal Society of London. Series B, Biological sciences, 364*(1532), 3093–3099. https://doi.org/10.1098/rstb.2009.0172

Reimers, S., & Dimmock, B. (1990). Mankind and kind men: an agenda for male family therapists. *Journal of Family Therapy, 12*(2), 167–181.

Scher, M. (1981). Men in hiding: a challenge for the counselor. *Personnel and Guidance Journal, 60*(4), 199–202.

Scott, S. (1998). Aggressive behaviour in childhood. *BMJ, 316*(7126), 202–206.

Sheppard, M. (2002). Mental health and social justice: Gender, race and psychological consequences of unfairness. *The British Journal of Social Work, 32*(6), 779–797. http:// www.jstor.org/stable/23716495

Slive, Z .S. (1986). The feminist therapist and the male client. *Women and Therapy, 5*(2–3), 81–87.

Snow, R. C. (2008). Sex, gender, and vulnerability. *Global Public Health 3* Suppl 1: 58–74. 10.1080/17441690801902619

Stangl, A. L., Earnshaw, V. A., Logie, C. H. *et al.* (2019). The health stigma and discrimination framework: a global, crosscutting framework to inform research, intervention development, and policy on health-related stigmas. *BMC Medicine, 17* (31). https:// doi.org/10.1186/s12916-019-1271-3

Tampi, R. R., Young, J., Hoq, R., Resnick, K., & Tampi, D. J. (2019). Psychotic disorders in late life: a narrative review. *Therapeutic Advances in Psychopharmacology, 9*, 2045125319882798. https://doi.org/10.1177/2045125319882798

Vlassoff, C. (1994). Gender inequalities in health in the Third World: uncharted ground. *Social Science & Medicine, 39*(9), 1249–1259.

Vlassoff, C., & Moreno, C. G. (2002). Placing gender at the center of health programming: challenges and limitations. *Social Science & Medicine, 54*(11), 1713–1723.

World Health Organization. (1998). *Gender and Health: Technical Paper* (No. WHO/FRH/ WHD/98.16.) . Geneva: World Health Organization.

World Health Organization. (2001). *Mental Health: New Understanding, New Hope*. Geneva: World Health Organization.

World Health Organization. (2006). *Gender and Women's Mental Health*. www.who.int/ mental_health/prevention/genderwomen/en/print.html.

World Health Organization (2011). Mental Health Atlas. http://apps.who.int/iris/ bitstream/10665/44697/1/9799241564359_eng.pdf.

Index

For Product Safety Concerns and Information please contact our EU
representative GPSR@taylorandfrancis.com
Taylor & Francis Verlag GmbH, Kaufingerstraße 24, 80331 München, Germany

9 780367 542054